Esophageal Disorders

Francisco Schlottmann
Fernando A. M. Herbella • Marco G. Patti
Editors

Esophageal Disorders

Diagnosis and Treatment

Springer

Editors
Francisco Schlottmann
University of Buenos Aires,
Ciudad Autónoma Buenos Aires
Buenos Aires, Argentina

Fernando A. M. Herbella
Department of Surgery
Federal University of São Paulo
São Paulo, São Paulo, Brazil

Marco G. Patti
Department of Surgery
University of Virginia Hospital
Charlottesville, VA, USA

ISBN 978-3-032-08178-0 ISBN 978-3-032-08179-7 (eBook)
https://doi.org/10.1007/978-3-032-08179-7

This Springer imprint is published by the registered company Springer Nature Switzerland AG
The registered company address is: Gewerbestrasse 11, 6330 Cham, Switzerland

To Dr. Marco G. Patti, life mentor who always provides guidance and support.
To Dr. Rudolf Buxhoeveden, who inspired me during my training to become a minimally invasive foregut surgeon.

Francisco Schlottmann

Among many surgeons that I crossed paths with and surely most of them taught me something, Dr. Marco Patti is the greatest of them

Fernando A.M. Herbella

To Francisco Schlottmann and Fernando Herbella, grateful for your friendship and collaboration over the years. My best wishes for a happy life and a fulfilling career.

Marco G. Patti

Contents

Esophageal Anatomy

Rafael C. Katayama, Fernando A. M. Herbella,
Francisco Schlottmann, and Marco G. Patti

Introduction

Some special features of the surgical anatomy of the esophagus should be summarized: (1) the major organs surround the esophagus, (2) the esophagus passes through the neck, chest and abdomen, (3) the esophagus is limited by sphincters, (4) the lymphatic distribution is abundant, and (5) the organs and structures of the mediastinum may often show anatomical variations [1]. Unfortunately, the classical anatomical description of some organs and structures differs from the clinical presentation. Anatomists frequently portrait the esophagus in didactic books in a stylized fashion commonly not useful for surgeons (Fig. 1). In addition, minimally invasive surgery also brought a restricted but magnified view of the esophagus, and available imaging technology forces the understanding of sectional and regional anatomy [3]. Sir William Halsted, father of the surgical residence training among other remarkable achievements, may be quoted regarding the view provided by dissecting a patient during surgery: there is a gap between the surgeon and the pathologist that only the surgeon can bridge. The pathologist rarely has the opportunity to see pathological conditions as the surgeon sees them. Furthermore, there is no standardization of classification and nomenclature of some structures in and around the esophagus [1].

R. C. Katayama · F. A. M. Herbella (✉)
Gastrointestinal Surgery - Esophagus and Stomach Division - Department of Surgery, Federal University of São Paulo, São Paulo, Brazil
e-mail: herbella.dcir@epm.br

F. Schlottmann
University of Buenos Aires, Ciudad Autónoma Buenos Aires, Buenos Aires, Argentina

M. G. Patti
Department of Surgery, University of Virginia Hospital, Charlottesville, VA, USA

F. Schlottmann et al. (eds.), *Esophageal Disorders*,
https://doi.org/10.1007/978-3-032-08179-7_1

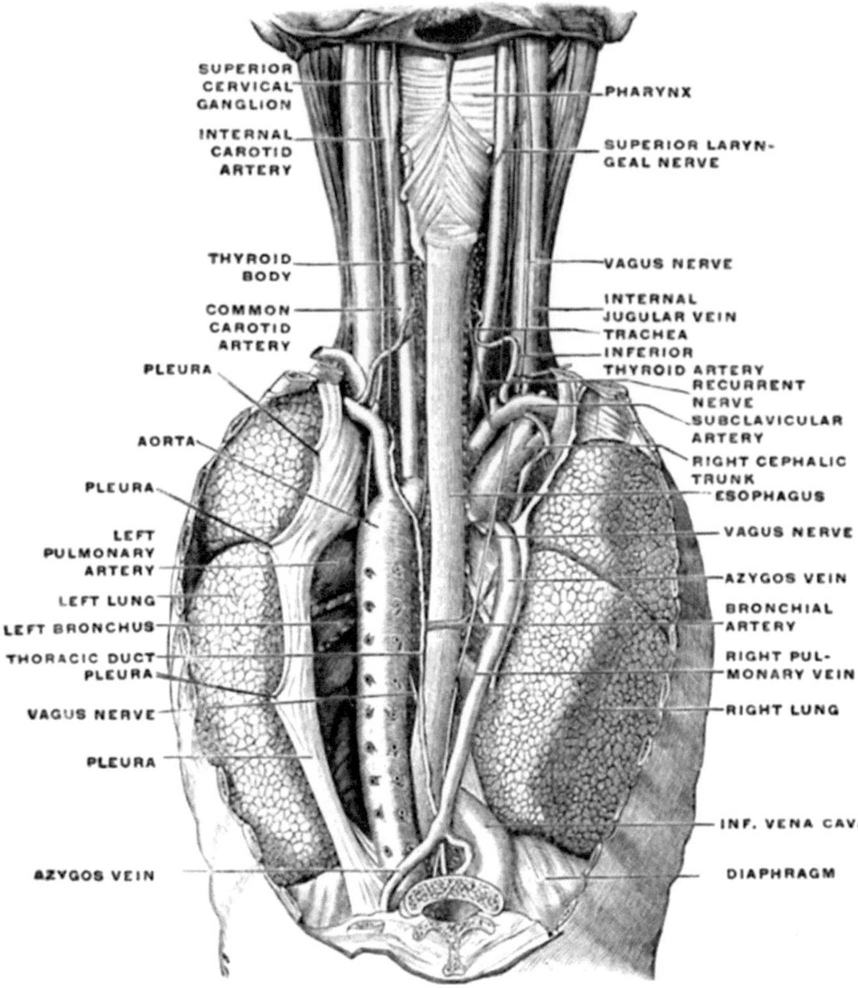

Fig. 1 The esophagus as represented in anatomy textbooks. (From Gray and Lewis [2]. Public domain)

Esophageal anatomy cannot be understood apart from esophageal physiology. Esophageal benign diseases, the scope of this book, are basically physiological diseases and mostly confined to the distal esophagus and esophagogastric junction. This chapter will focus on this area.

Esophageal Anatomy

The esophagus is a hollow tubular organ with similar layers of other digestive organs (mucosa, submucosa, muscularis propria) except for the serosa that is replaced by an adventitia [4]. Also different from other digestive organs, skeletal muscle forms the upper third of the esophageal musculature and smooth muscle the lower two thirds. The esophagus has 3 parts: cervical, thoracic, and abdominal. The thoracic portion may also be subdivided in: (a) Upper thoracic esophagus—from the sternal notch to the tracheal bifurcation; (b) Middle thoracic esophagus—the proximal half of the two equal portions between the tracheal bifurcation and the esophagogastric junction; and (c) Lower thoracic esophagus—the thoracic part of the distal half of the two equal portions between the tracheal bifurcation and the esophagogastric junction [5].

Esophageal blood supply comes from branches of the inferior thyroid arteries, thoracic aorta, bronchial arteries, inferior phrenic arteries, and left gastric artery. Blood drains into the inferior thyroid, hemiazygos, azygos, and left gastric veins. There is not a dedicated vessel to the esophagus [6]. Abundant lymphatics form a dense submucosal plexus [5].

Textbook Anatomy

Figure 2 depicts diagrammatically the esophagus and surrounding anatomy. The cervical portion may be the center for esophagopharyngeal diverticula (Zenker and Killian). Surgical anatomy of the thoracic esophagus is of major interest for oncologic diseases of the esophagus. The abdominal esophagus and distal part of the thoracic are the center for most benign diseases of the esophagus within interest of surgeons.

Cadaveric Anatomy

Esophageal anatomy learned in anatomy laboratories is the clear definition of the gap between the surgeon and the pathologist. Not different form schematic drawings, it does not reflect the complexity of surgical access to this posterior organ surrounded by important structures. It also does not reflect the distortion in anatomy caused by a large hiatal hernia, e.g. (Fig. 3)

Surgical anatomy in fresh cadavers (Fig. 4) may have a good resemblance to real situation and are a good model for experimentation [7] and teaching [8].

Radiologic Anatomy

Barium esophagram (Fig. 5) is able to provide a panoramic view of the esophagus. Despite the resemblance of an anatomic model in which the relation between the esophagus and other structures is not really clear, the test has the advantage of a physiological interpretation of the anatomy [9].

Computed tomography (Fig. 6)/magnetic resonance are important to show spaces not understood by the naked eye during an operation and relations with other organs. This has advantages for the study of complications after esophageal operations.

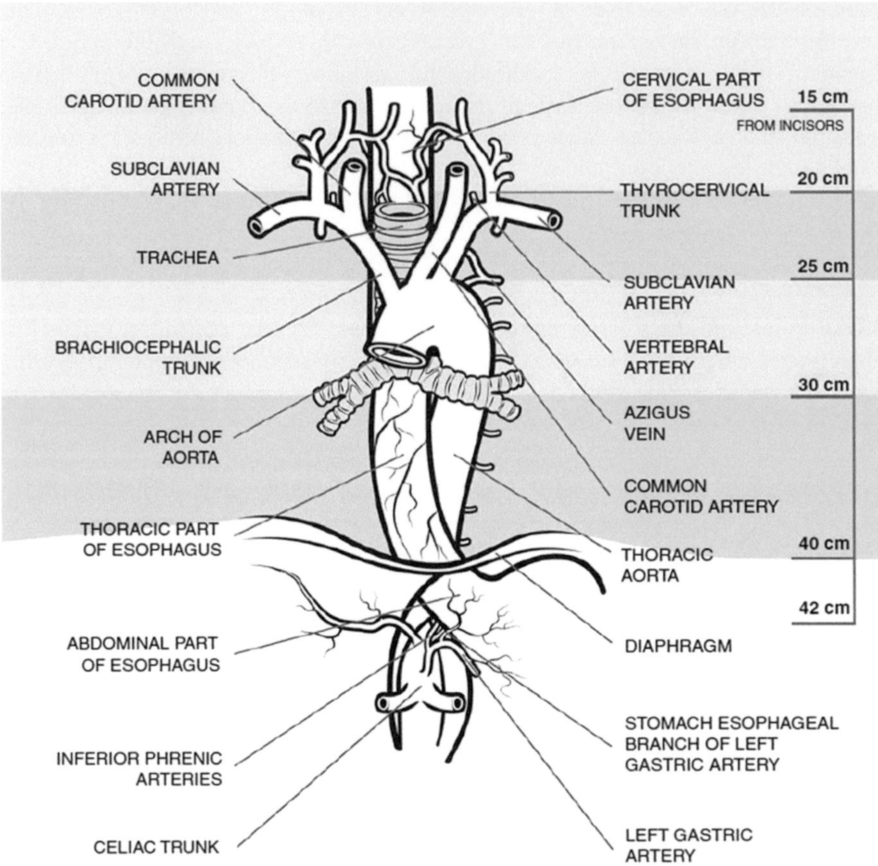

Fig. 2 Esophageal anatomy: the three portions of the esophagus and surrounding structures in the posterior mediastinum. (Reproduced from: Menezes et al. [3])

They are; however, not functional tests, although some attempts to evaluate physiology have been tried but never gained popularity [10]. Three-dimension images (Fig. 7) are opening a new understanding of the anatomy that may help surgeons in surgical planning [11].

Intraoperative Anatomy

Mostly of the operations for benign esophageal diseases are currently performed through the laparoscopic route [12]. This route provides a magnified but restricted view of the anatomy. This view may be quite different from the naked eye open approach (Fig. 8).

In order to reach the esophagogastric junction, that is the center for most esophageal benign disease operations, the gastrohepatic ligamentum of the lesser

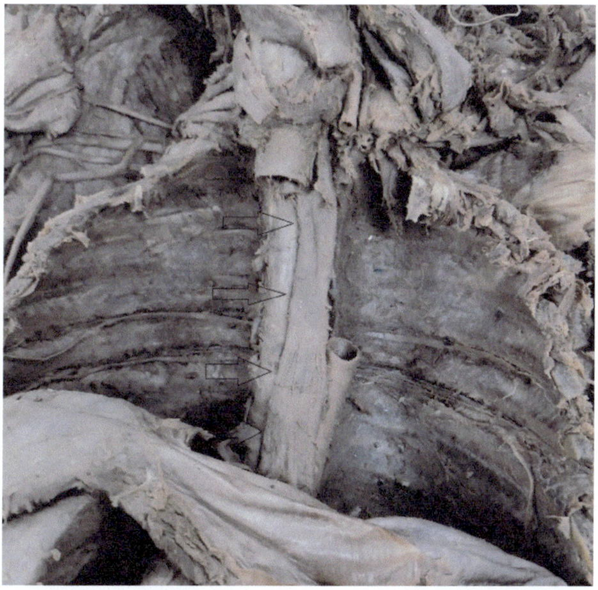

Fig. 3 The anatomy of the esophagus (arrows) as seen in dissected embalmed cadavers

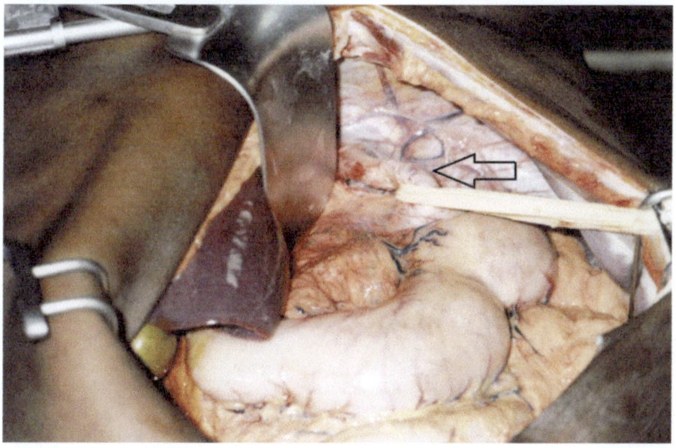

Fig. 4 Dissection of the abdominal part of the esophagus (arrow) in fresh cadavers simulating a real open operation

omentum must be divided. It contains the hepatic branch of the vagus nerve and occasionally an accessory hepatic branch from the left gastric artery. Both structures may be divided with impunity. The opened ligament will show the caudate lobe of the liver, the right pillar of the right crus of the esophageal hiatus and the phrenoesophageal membrane encircling the esophagus. Dissection of the membrane will show the distal esophagus (distal portion of the thoracic esophagus and the abdominal portion) [14]. The anterior vagus nerve is usually branched, close to the esophagus and more to the left side. The posterior vagus nerve is, oppositely, a unique trunk, detached from the esophagus and more to the right side.

Fig. 5 Barium swallow esophagram showing the contrasted esophagus (arrow)

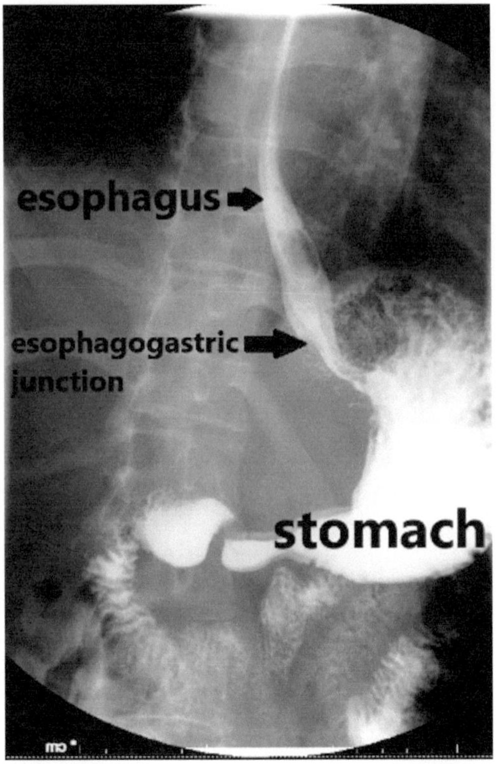

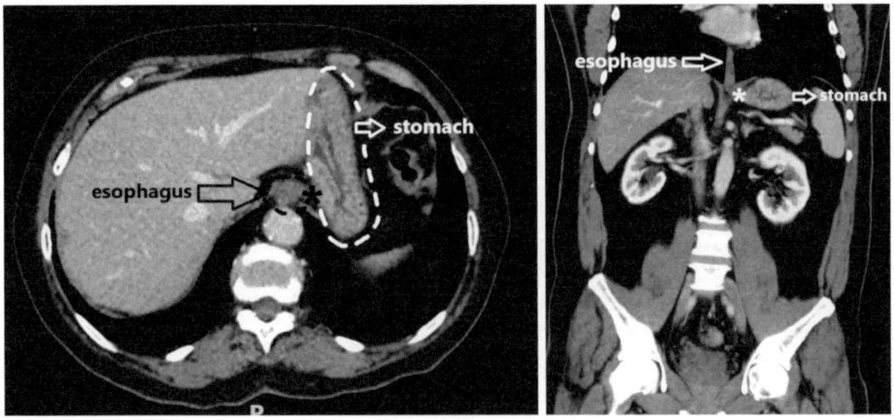

Fig. 6 Computed tomography imaging of the esophagus and esophagogastric junction (*)

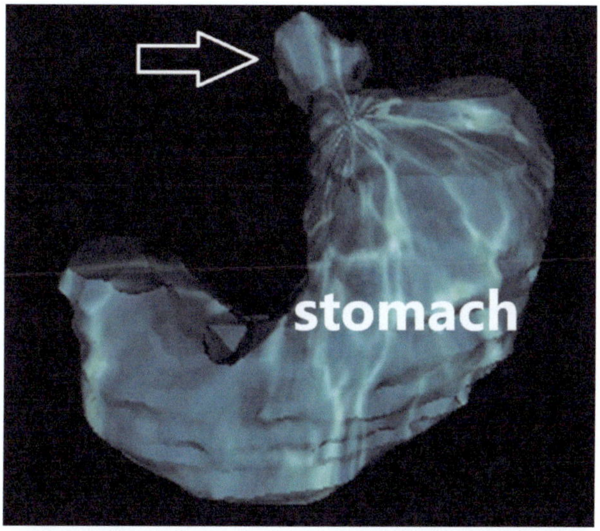

Fig. 7 Three-dimensional computed tomography imaging of the distal esophagus (arrow)

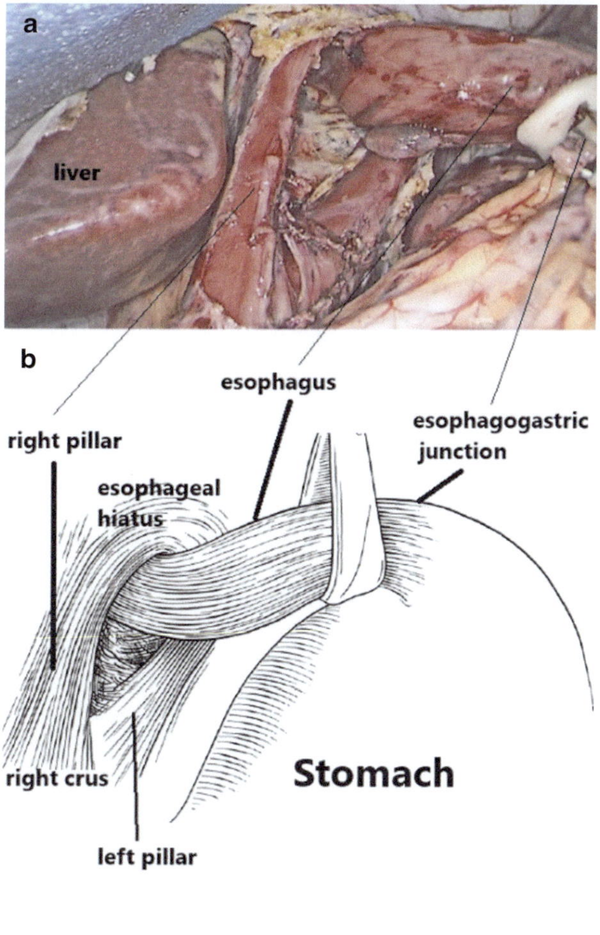

Fig. 8 Laparoscopic view of the esophagogastric junction area. (Adapted from Patti et al. [13])

The Boundaries of the Esophagus

The definitions of the boundaries of the esophagus are of key importance to define hiatal hernia and to guide surgeons during operations that need to perfectly identify the esophagogastric junction.

The upper esophageal sphincter marks the upper border of the esophagus. It is formed by the cricopharyngeus muscle along with the inferior constrictors of the pharynx and fibers of the esophageal wall. It corresponds to the pharyngoesophageal transition just posterior to the cricoid cartilage, that has a clear superficial anatomy view, and it is easily palpated. This parameter may guide incisions aimed at this area.

The lower border of the esophagus is variable considering how it is defined. Moreover, a hiatal hernia is defined by the presence of the esophagogastric junction (or part of the stomach in case of paraesophageal hernias) above the diaphragm, but the diaphragm, is seen by different parameters in distinct situations. Provocative tests forcing the stomach upwards are also variable according to the situation. This may explain discrepancy in different tests showing hiatal hernia or not or different measurements.

Physiologically, as measured by esophageal manometry e.g., the lower border corresponds to the lower esophageal sphincter (LES) that is not a separate anatomic structure but a physiological valvular mechanism. The diaphragm is noticed as phasic contractions [15]. Provocative maneuvers may be applied such as leg raising [16].

During an operation, the transition from the tubular to a sacular organ, the angle of His, and the transition from exposed muscular fibers denoting the absence of a serosa to the bright serosa of the stomach mark the esophagogastric junction. The diaphragm is seen as the crus surrounding the esophagus. Anesthesia with muscular blockade may relax the diaphragm and abdominal wall forcing viscera down to the abdomen. On the other hand, pneumoperitoneum may push viscera up.

Endoscopically, the lower border of the esophagus is seen as the epithelial transition (Z line) and the diaphragm as an extrinsic constriction at or distal do the transition (Fig. 9). Gastric insufflation with air and superficial sedation may contribute to upwards displacement of the stomach [17].

Radiologically, the esophagogastric junction is defined by the transition from the tubular esophagus to the sacular stomach, as previously shown at the esophagram and computerized tomography. Provocative maneuvers such as Trendelenburg position and abdominal compression may be used to displace viscera upwards.

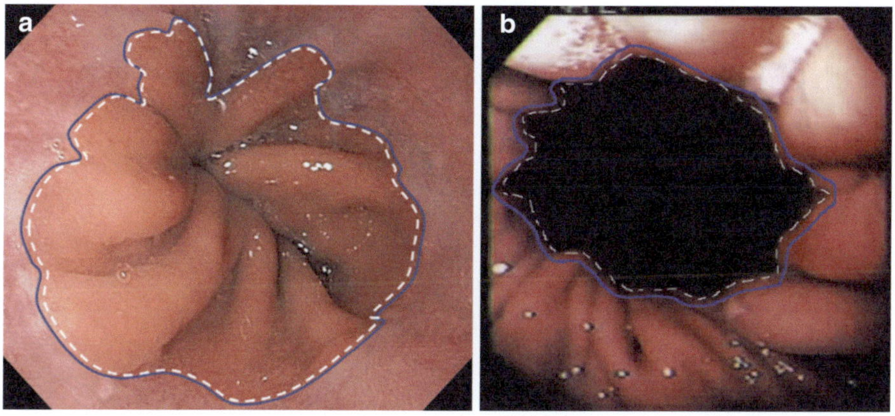

Fig. 9 Endoscopic parameters for the esophagogastric junction—epithelial transition (**a**—lines) and the diaphragm—extrinsic constriction (**b**—lines)

Functional Anatomy

The negative thoracic pressure and the positive abdominal pressure leads to a transdiaphragmatic pressure gradient between the esophagus and the stomach. This gradient would lead inexorably to the reflux of gastric contents into the esophagus if not by the presence of a valvular mechanism at the level of the esophagogastric junction (EGJ). Despite the existence of this barrier, gastroesophageal reflux disease (GERD) is very common [18].

The Antireflux Barrier Components

The anatomical arrangement of the LES, hiatus, angle of His and phrenoesophageal ligaments forms the anti-reflux barrier (Fig. 10).

The Lower Esophageal Sphincter

The LES is a circular smooth muscle that is tonically contracted at rest, creating a high-pressure zone in the distal esophagus. It extends 2–3 cm above the squamous columnar mucosal junction, and its distal margin is about 2 cm below this junction. The upper part lies at the level of the diaphragmatic crura, while the lower part is intra-abdominal under abdominal pressure. The LES measures approximately 2.5–4.5 cm in length and consists of different muscle fibers (circular, oblique, and sling) with varying physiological traits, resulting in an asymmetrical pressure pattern. The LES is the main component of the anti-reflux barrier, it is able to maintain its function even when all other components are absent, as in patients with hiatal hernia without GERD [19].

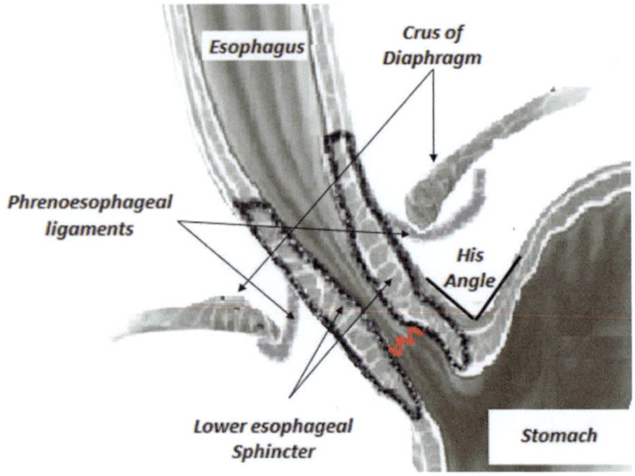

Fig. 10 Components of the gastroesophageal antireflux barrier. (Reproduced from Del Grande et al. [19])

Crural Diaphragm

The LES lies in a hiatus created by the right crus of the diaphragm and is supported by phrenoesophageal ligaments. This, along with the basal pressure of the sphincter, creates a high-pressure zone seen in manometry. The diaphragmatic crus pinches the LES, contributing to resting pressure and keeping it in position. Crural diaphragm contraction increases esophagogastric pressure during abdominal straining and compression [20].

Phrenoesophageal Membrane

The visceral peritoneum and the phrenoesophageal membrane keep the esophagogastric in the abdominal cavity. Phrenoesophageal ligaments are a fibrous connective tissue extending from the muscle fibers of the diaphragm to the distal portion of the esophagus. The membrane extends 2–3 cm above the hiatus, transmitting the positive abdominal pressure to the distal esophagus [20, 21].

Angle of His

The acute angle formed between the esophagus and the gastric fundus (angle of His) creates a longer distance between where the food is stored (the gastric fundus) and the esophagus where it can reflux. Also, the apex of this angle creates the *Gubaroff valves* or *plica cardiaca,* a cushion fold of the mucosa at the level of the esophagogastric junction acting as a stopper [22].

References

1. Takassi GF, Herbella FA, Patti MG. Variações anatômicas na anatomia cirúrgica do esôfago torácico e suas estruturas circundantes [Anatomic variations in the surgical anatomy of the thoracic esophagus and its surrounding structures]. Arq Bras Cir Dig. 2013;26(2):101–6. Portuguese. https://doi.org/10.1590/s0102-67202013000200006.

2. Gray H, Lewis WH. Anatomy of the human body. 2nd ed. Philadelphia, New York: Lea & Febiger; 1924.
3. Menezes MA, Sato RO, Schlottmann F, Herbella FAM. Esophageal anatomy. In: Schlottmann F, Molena D, Patti M, editors. Esophageal cancer. Cham: Springer; 2018. p. 1–13. https://doi.org/10.1007/978-3-319-91830-3_1.
4. Rice TW, Bronner MP. The esophageal wall. Thorac Surg Clin. 2011;21(2):299–305. https://doi.org/10.1016/j.thorsurg.2011.01.005.
5. Menezes MA, Sato RO, Schlottmann F, Herbella FA. Esophageal anatomy. In: Schlottmann F, Molena D, Patti MG, editors. Esophageal cancer: diagnosis and treatment. Springer; 2018. p. 1–13.
6. Patti MG, Gantert W, Way LW. Surgery of the esophagus. Anatomy and physiology. Surg Clin North Am. 1997;77(5):959–70.
7. Herbella FA, Del Grande JC. Human cadavers as an experimental model for esophageal surgery. Dis Esophagus. 2001;14(3–4):218–22. https://doi.org/10.1046/j.1442-2050.2001.00205.x.
8. Herbella FA. Are surgeons too far from the anatomy lab? Contemp Surg. 2004;60(2):64.
9. Andolfi C, Vigneswaran Y, Kavitt RT, Herbella FA, Patti MG. Laparoscopic antireflux surgery: importance of patient's selection and preoperative workup. J Laparoendosc Adv Surg Tech A. 2017;27(2):101–5. https://doi.org/10.1089/lap.2016.0322.
10. Covotta F, Piretta L, Badiali D, Laghi A, Biondi T, Corazziari ES, Panebianco V. Functional magnetic resonance in the evaluation of oesophageal motility disorders. Gastroenterol Res Pract. 2011;2011:367639. https://doi.org/10.1155/2011/367639.
11. Santana AV, Herbella FAM, Domene CE, Volpe P, Neto WCGM, Polízio RP, Tamamoto FD, Katayama RC, Patti MG. High-resolution 3-dimensional tomography may be a useful tool for understanding the anatomy of hiatal hernias and surgical planning of patients eligible for laparoscopic or robotic antireflux surgery. Surg Endosc. 2024;38(2):780–6. https://doi.org/10.1007/s00464-023-10599-5.
12. Bello B, Herbella FA, Allaix ME, Patti MG. Impact of minimally invasive surgery on the treatment of benign esophageal disorders. World J Gastroenterol. 2012;18(46):6764–70. https://doi.org/10.3748/wjg.v18.i46.6764.
13. Patti MG, Schlottmann B, Herbella FAM, Borraez B. Operations for gastroesophageal reflux disease. In: Herbella FAM, Patti MG, editors. Atlas of esophageal surgery. 2nd ed. New York: Springer; 2022. p. 45–62.
14. Kuster GG, Innocenti FA. Laparoscopic anatomy of the region of the esophageal hiatus. Surg Endosc. 1997;11(9):883–93. https://doi.org/10.1007/s004649900480.
15. Dias NCB, Herbella FAM, Del Grande LM, Patti MG. The transdiaphragmatic pressure gradient and the lower esophageal sphincter in the pathophysiology of gastroesophageal reflux disease: an analysis of 500 esophageal function tests. J Gastrointest Surg. 2023;27(4):677–81. https://doi.org/10.1007/s11605-022-05529-0.
16. Rim DS, Parkman HP. Comparative evaluation of single versus double leg raise maneuver in high-resolution esophageal manometry. Neurogastroenterol Motil. 2024;36(10):e14868. https://doi.org/10.1111/nmo.14868.
17. Tolone S, Savarino E, Zaninotto G, Gyawali CP, Frazzoni M, de Bortoli N, Frazzoni L, Del Genio G, Bodini G, Furnari M, Savarino V, Docimo L. High-resolution manometry is superior to endoscopy and radiology in assessing and grading sliding hiatal hernia: a comparison with surgical in vivo evaluation. United European Gastroenterol J. 2018;6(7):981–9. https://doi.org/10.1177/2050640618769160.
18. Del Grande LM, Herbella FAM, Katayama RC, Schlottmann F, Patti MG. The role of the transdiaphragmatic pressure gradient in the pathophysiology of gastroesophageal reflux disease. Arq Gastroenterol. 2018;55(Suppl 1):13–7. https://doi.org/10.1590/S0004-2803.201800000-39.
19. Del Grande LM, Figueiredo FBP, Herbella FAM, Schlottmann F, Patti MG. Esophageal anatomy: the antireflux barrier. In: Schlottmann F, Patti MG, Herbella FAM, editors. Gastroesophageal reflux disease. From pathophysiology to treatment. Springer; 2024. p. 1–6.

20. Holloway RH. The anti-reflux barrier and mechanisms of gastro-oesophageal reflux. Baillieres Best Pract Res Clin Gastroenterol. 2000;14(5):681–99. https://doi.org/10.1053/bega.2000.0118.
21. Michelson E, Siegel CI. The role of the phrenico-esophageal ligament in the lower esophageal sphincter. Surg Gynecol Obstet. 1964;118:1291–4.
22. Menezes MA, Herbella FAM. Pathophysiology of gastroesophageal reflux disease. World J Surg. 2017;41(7):1666–71. https://doi.org/10.1007/s00268-017-3952-4.

Pathophysiology of Gastroesophageal Reflux Disease

Rafael C. Katayama, Fernando A. M. Herbella, Marco G. Patti, and Francisco Schlottmann

Introduction

Gastroesophageal reflux disease (GERD) is a highly prevalent disease, especially in Western countries. Its pathophysiology is complex and multifactorial. It occurs when the intricate valve mechanism at the level of the esophagogastric junction (EGJ) is not capable of balancing the transdiaphragmatic pressure gradient (positive intra-abdominal pressure and negative intra-thoracic pressure) leading to the return of food and gastric content to the esophagus [1, 2].

Although the intricate valvular mechanism is quite efficient, a small amount of reflux is considered normal and balanced by the salivary production and esophageal clearance promoted by esophageal peristalsis [3, 4]. In the other hand, the lower esophageal sphincter (LES), the diaphragm, the angle of His, the Gubaroff valve and the phrenoesophageal membrane act together to compose the valvular mechanism, responsible for the barrier at the level of EGJ [3]. When this barrier is not capable of balance the transdiaphragmatic pressure, food, acid and bile rises into the esophagus. The chemical damage to esophageal mucosa is responsible for esophageal injury associated with GERD symptoms [2]. Chemical aggression leads to mucosal inflammation, breaking up the tight junction proteins of the esophageal epithelium, resulting in increased para-cellular permeability and dilated intercellular space. Consequently, gastric acid, bile, and pepsin penetrate deep basal

R. C. Katayama (✉) · F. A. M. Herbella
Department of Surgery, Escola Paulista de Medicina, Federal University of São Paulo, São Paulo, Brazil
e-mail: Caue.katayama@unifesp.br

M. G. Patti
Department of Surgery, University of Virginia Hospital, Charlottesville, VA, USA

F. Schlottmann
University of Buenos Aires, Ciudad Autónoma Buenos Aires, Buenos Aires, Argentina

F. Schlottmann et al. (eds.), *Esophageal Disorders*,
https://doi.org/10.1007/978-3-032-08179-7_2

layers of the esophageal mucosa stimulating inflammatory mediators [5, 6]. This inflammation is responsible for esophageal dysmotility and GERD symptoms [7, 8].

Natural Anti-reflux Mechanism

1. **Peristalsis**

When chemical elements rises to the esophagus, the longer they remain in contact with the mucosa, the greater the damage will be done. Esophagus clearance secondary to peristalsis is an important mechanism to prevent mucosal damage. Defective peristalsis is associated with GERD symptoms and mucosal damage, related to the time of exposure of esophageal mucosa to chemical agents (acid, bile and pepsine) [3].

It is common that patients with GERD have abnormal peristalsis because of the inflammation of the esophagus. The severity of this dysmotility is related to abnormal propagation of peristaltic waves (ineffective esophageal motility) and/or an extremely low amplitude of peristalsis. If esophageal clearance is compromised, the contact time of the refluxate increases, resulting in greater severity of the GERD. Possibly this fact may facilitate reflux to the upper esophagus and pharynx. Therefore, these patients are at greater risk for severe mucosal lesions and frequent extraesophageal symptoms [9–12].

2. **Lower esophageal sphincter**

One of the main components of the valve intricate mechanism is LES. The LES is a muscle, 3–4 cm in length, located at the distal end of the esophagus. Its function is to allow the passage of food into the gastric chamber by relaxing its fibers coordinated with esophagus peristalsis. Also, allowing gas venting after meals and preventing reflux of gastric contents by returning to its initial tonus, pressuring the transition of the esophagus to the stomach [13]. An effective LES must have an adequate total and intra-abdominal length, and resting pressure. A defective LES is found in most patients with GERD; however, it is not an essential condition. It is known that normal LES pressure can be found in 40% of patients with GERD. Although this apparent inconsistency, it can be understood because transient LES relaxations (TLSER) may influence GERD. TSLER are defined as LES relaxations, lasting at least 10 s that occur in the absence of swallowing and can be the genesis of pathological reflux [14, 15]. Furthermore, an increase transdiaphragmatic pressure gradient should overcome the LES mechanism promoting pathological reflux, mainly in patients with increasing abdominal pressure (obesity) or more negative thoracic pressure (pulmonary disease) [16].

3. **Angle of His**

The angle of His is an acute angle formed by the esophagus and the gastric fundus. This acute angle provides a barrier to the refluxate enlarging the distance between the gastric fundus, where food is stored, and the EGJ. The more acute the angle, the longer is the distance between the gastric fundus and more effective should be this barrier [3].

4. **Diaphragm and intra-abdominal esophagus length**

The diaphragmatic crus act reenforcing LES mechanism. It pinches the abdominal part of the esophagus at the level of the EGJ adding pressure to the LES, being part of an extrinsic component of the gastroesophageal barrier [3, 10].

The intra-abdominal portion of the esophagus receives influence of abdominal pressure that may help in the valve mechanism while collapsing the distal esophagus wall. A hiatus hernia breaks this mechanism due to the rise of EGJ to the thorax, placing it in a negative pressure regime [17–19].

5. **Gubaroff Valve**

Gubaroff valves consist of a cushion action of the distal esophageal mucosa at the level of the EGJ [20, 21].

Transdiaphragmatic Pressure

The transdiaphragmatic pressure consists in the gradient between forces acting in the abdomen and thorax. The abdominal pressure tends to be positive pushing gastric content toward thorax. In the other hand, the thoracic pressure tends to be negative, generating suction of the gastric content. However, this gradient is normally balanced by natural valvular mechanisms [22, 23], except in situations when an increase in the abdominal pressure or a decrease in the thoracic pressure overcomes the valvular mechanism [24].

Special Clinical Conditions and GERD

A. **Thoracic pressure and GERD**

An increased respiratory effort may lead to more negative thoracic pressure. This condition can be seen in singers, professional wind instrument players or patients with obstructive pulmonary diseases. The decrease in thoracic pressure should influence transdiaphragmatic pressure, consequently rising the incidence of GERD [25, 26].

B. **Abdominal pressure and GERD**

Elevated abdominal pressure is one of the most important independent risk factors for GERD development. The most prevalent clinical condition associated with the rise in intraabdominal pressure is obesity. Abdominal fat deposition and abdominal circumference are directly related to the rise of abdominal pressure [16, 24, 27].

Although an increased basal LES pressure can be observed in patients with obesity, probably secondary to a compensatory mechanism to overcome the elevated intraabdominal pressure, TSLER seems to be more frequent in this clinical condition. Therefore, the higher incidence of TSLER will lead to an increase in GERD prevalence [24, 28].

Another important concern is that patients with obesity have a decrease in salivation and esophageal motility may be impaired in 25% of patients with this condition. Moreover, the fat deposition in the EGJ can make this angle obtuse, worsening the valvular mechanism [24].

Patients with obesity may also have decreased intrathoracic pressure related to the higher incidence of obstructive apnea. Besides that, patients with this condition could have an elevation in the diaphragm, consequently decreasing the pulmonary expansion, reflecting in the thoracic pressure. This association is responsible for the disruption of the valvular mechanism, therefore, increasing the risk of GERD [29, 30].

C. **Hiatal Hernia and GERD**

Hiatal Hernia (HH) can disrupt most of antireflux barrier mechanisms. However, GERD and HH are not synonyms. Actually, it is well known that those conditions can exist independently [31]. But this association is justified because HH enlarges the hiatus, losing the pinchcock action of the diaphragm, leading to a more incompetent LES, defective peristalsis, more severe mucosal damage, and increased acid exposure. Moreover, when the esophagus rises toward the thorax the angle of His is disrupted and the abdominal pressure is no more effective in the distal esophagus, impairing the valvular mechanism. Finally, TLESR is more frequent in patients with hiatal hernia [32, 33].

D. **Dysmotility and GERD**

Ineffective esophageal motility may be present in a quarter of patients with GERD. Esophageal peristalsis is a central mechanism for esophagus clearance. Primary esophageal dysmotility should decrease clearance and be responsible for mucosa damage. On the other hand, GERD is responsible for esophageal inflammation, consequently affecting esophageal peristalsis. Between this and that, it is not clear who comes first. However, studies could demonstrate an improvement in esophageal motility after reflux control with a surgical fundoplication [34, 35].

E. **Barret's Esophagus**

Gastric acid is recognized as very harmful to esophageal mucosa. However, gastroesophageal refluxate may contain other noxious agents as bile and pancreatic enzymes coming from duodenum. It is known that this component of the refluxate should damage esophageal mucosa and are also responsible for Barret's development and ultimately esophageal adenocarcinoma [36, 37].

F. **Sleeve Gastrectomy**

Sleeve Gastrectomy (SG) is one of the most performed bariatric procedures worldwide.

However, anatomical changes inherent to the procedure may favor GERD development. Stapling near the EGJ disrupts the Angle of His and may harm the muscle fibers of LES increasing TRLES. The phrenoesophageal membrane is damaged, impairing the extrinsic component of the gastroesophageal barrier. Finally, the Gastric Pouch after SG is a narrow-pressurized tube which may influence the trans-diaphragmatic pressure [38].

Conclusions

GERD pathophysiology is complex and multifactorial. GERD will be present when a disbalance between the intrinsic valvular mechanism (Table 1) and the transdiaphragmatic pressure gradient occurs. Specific clinical conditions (Table 2) such as obesity, hiatal hernia, Sleeve Gastrectomy, esophageal dysmotility and obstructive pulmonary diseases may affect this balance. Accordingly, it is crucial to understand GERD pathophysiology and special clinical conditions in order to provide the best treatment.

Table 1 Natural anti-reflux barrier

1. Peristalsis	Esophagus clearance secondary to peristalsis is an important mechanism to prevent mucosal damage.
2. Lower esophageal sphincter	A muscle, 3–4 cm in length, located at the distal end of the esophagus. Its function is to allow the passage of food into the gastric chamber by relaxing its fibers coordinated with esophagus peristalsis, avoiding reflux.
3. Angle of His	An acute angle formed by the esophagus and the gastric fundus. This acute angle provides a barrier to the refluxate enlarging the distance between the gastric fundus, where food is stored, and the esophagus gastric junction.
4. Diaphragm	It pinches the abdominal part of the esophagus at the level of esophagus gastric junction adding pressure to the lower esophageal sphincter.
5. Intra-abdominal esophagus length	The intra-abdominal portion of the esophagus receives the influence of abdominal pressure that may help in the valve mechanism while collapsing the distal esophagus wall.
6. Gubaroff valve	Consists of a cushion action of the distal esophageal mucosa at the level of the esophagus gastric junction.

Table 2 Special conditions that may influence GERD

Increased abdominal pressure	Decreased thoracic pressure	Failed valve mechanism
Obesity (abdominal fat) Singers Wind instrument players Pregnancy	Obstructive apnea Chronic pulmonary obstruction disease Asthma	Hiatal hernia Hypotonic lower esophageal sphincter Sleeve gastrectomy

References

1. Herbella FAM, Schlottmann F, Patti MG. Pathophysiology of gastroesophageal reflux disease: how an antireflux procedure works (or does not work). Updates Surg. 2018;70(3):343–7. https://doi.org/10.1007/s13304-018-0562-0. Epub 2018 Jul 23.
2. Menezes MA, Herbella FAM. Pathophysiology of gastroesophageal reflux disease. World J Surg. 2017;41(7):1666–71. https://doi.org/10.1007/s00268-017-3952-4.
3. Herbella FA, Patti MG. Gastroesophageal reflux disease: from pathophysiology to treatment. World J Gastroenterol. 2010;16(30):3745–9. https://doi.org/10.3748/wjg.v16.i30.3745. PMID: 20698035; PMCID: PMC2921084.
4. Patti MG, Vela MF, Odell DD, Richter JE, Fisichella PM, Vaezi MF. The intersection of GERD, aspiration, and lung transplantation. J Laparoendosc Adv Surg Tech A. 2016;26(7):501–5. 1670 World J Surg (2017) 41:1666–1671 123.
5. Ustaoglu A, Nguyen A, Spechler S, Sifrim D, Souza R, Woodland P. Mucosal pathogenesis in gastro-esophageal reflux disease. Neurogastroenterol Motil. 2020;32(12):e14022. https://doi.org/10.1111/nmo.14022. Epub 2020 Oct 28.
6. Miwa H, Kondo T, Oshima T. Gastroesophageal reflux disease-related and functional heartburn: pathophysiology and treatment. Curr Opin Gastroenterol. 2016;32:344–52.
7. Mittal R, Vaezi MF. Esophageal motility disorders and gastroesophageal reflux disease. N Engl J Med. 2020;383(20):1961–72. https://doi.org/10.1056/NEJMra2000328.
8. Su A, Gandhy R, Barlow C, Triadaflopoulos G. Clinical and manometric characteristics of patients with Parkinson's disease and esophageal symptoms. Dis Esophagus. 2017;30(4):1–6.
9. Herbella FA, Tedesco P, Nipomnick I, Fisichella PM, Patti MG. Efect of partial and total laparoscopic fundoplication on esophageal body motility. Surg Endosc. 2007;21(2):285–8.
10. Patti MG, Gasper WJ, Fisichella PM, Nipomnick I, Palazzo F. Gastroesophageal reflux disease and connective tissue disorders: pathophysiology and implications for treatment. J Gastrointest Surg. 2008;12:1900–6.
11. Johnson LF, Demeester TR. Twenty-four-hour pH monitoring of the distal esophagus. A quantitative measure of gastroesophageal reflux. Am J Gastroenterol. 1974;62:325–32.
12. Xu JY, Xie XP, Song GQ, Hou XH. Healing of severe reflux esophagitis with PPI does not improve esophageal dysmotility. Dis Esophagus. 2007;20:346–52.
13. Hershcovici T, Mashimo H, Fass R. The lower esophageal sphincter. Neurogastroenterol Motil. 2011;23(9):819–30.
14. Benati CD, Herbella FA, Patti MG. Manometric parameters in patients with suspected gastroesophageal reflux disease and normal pH monitoring. GED Gastroenterol Endosc Dig. 2014;33(2):52–7.
15. Kahrilas PJ, Shi G, Manka M, Joehl RJ. Increased frequency of transient lower esophageal sphincter relaxation induced by gastric distention in reflux patients with hiatal hernia. Gastroenterology. 2000;118(4):688–95.
16. Del Grande LM, Herbella FA, Bigatao AM, Abrao H, Jardim JR, Patti MG. Pathophysiology of gastroesophageal refux in patients with chronic pulmonary obstructive disease is linked to an increased transdiaphragmatic pressure gradient and not to a defective esophagogastric barrier. J Gastrointest Surg. 2016;20(1):104–10.

17. Franzén T, Tibbling L. Is the severity of gastroesophageal reflux dependent on hiatus hernia size? World J Gastroenterol. 2014;20(6):1582–4.
18. Allison PR. Hiatus hernia: (a 20-year retrospective survey). Ann Surg. 1973;178(3):273–6.
19. Herbella FA. Secrets for successful laparoscopic antireflux surgery. Ann Laparosc Endosc Surg. 2017;2:46.
20. DeMeester TR, Wernly JA, Bryant GH, Little AG, Skinner DB. Clinical and in vitro analysis of determinants of gastroesophageal competence. A study of the principles of antirefux surgery. Am J Surg. 1979;137(1):39–46.
21. Valezi AC, Herbella FAM, Schlottmann F, Patti MG. Gastroesophageal reflux disease in obese patients. J Laparoendosc Adv Surg Tech A. 2018;28(8):949–52. https://doi.org/10.1089/lap.2018.0395. Epub 2018 Jul 13.
22. Gourcerol G, Benanni Y, Boueyre E, Leroi AM, Ducrotte P. Infuence of gastric emptying on gastro-esophageal reflux: a combined pH-impedance study. Neurogastroenterol Motil. 2013;25(10):800. https://doi.org/10.1111/nmo.12181.
23. Pregun I, Bakucz T, Banai J, et al. Gastroesophageal reflux disease: work-related disease? Dig Dis. 2009;27(1):38–44. https://doi.org/10.1159/000210102. (Epub 2009 May 8).
24. Nadaleto BF, Herbella FA, Patti MG. Gastroesophageal reflux disease in the obese: pathophysiology and treatment. Surgery. 2016;159(2):475–86.
25. Sweet MP, Herbella FA, Leard L, Hoopes C, Golden J, Hays S, Patti MG. The prevalence of distal and proximal gastroesophageal reflux in patients awaiting lung transplantation. Ann Surg. 2006;244:491–7.
26. Gasper WJ, Sweet MP, Hoopes C, Leard LE, Kleinhenz ME, Hays SR, Golden JA, Patti MG. Antirefux surgery for patients with end-stage lung disease before and after lung transplantation. Surg Endosc. 2008;22(2):495–50.
27. Felinska E, Billeter A, Nickel F, Contin P, Berlth F, Chand B, Grimminger P, Mikami D, Schoppmann SF, Müller-Stich B. Do we understand the pathophysiology of GERD after sleeve gastrectomy? Ann N Y Acad Sci. 2020;1482(1):26–35. https://doi.org/10.1111/nyas.14467. Epub 2020 Sep 6.
28. Schlottmann F, Dreifuss NH, Patti MG. Obesity and esophageal cancer: GERD, Barrett's esophagus, and molecular carcinogenic pathways. Expert Rev Gastroenterol Hepatol. 2020;14(6):425–33. https://doi.org/10.1080/17474124.2020.1764348. Epub 2020 May 22.
29. Herbella FA, Andolf C, Vigneswaran Y, Patti MG, Pinna BR. Importance of esophageal manometry and pH monitoring for the evaluation of otorhinolaryngologic (ENT) manifestations of GERD. A multicenter study. J Gastrointest Surg. 2016;20(10):1673–8. https://doi.org/10.1007/s11605-016-3212-1.
30. Herbella FA, Sweet MP, Tedesco P, Nipomnick I, Patti MG. Gastroesophageal reflux disease and obesity. Pathophysiology and implications for treatment. J Gastrointest Surg. 2007;11(3):286–90.
31. Stylopoulos N, Rattner DW. The history of hiatal hernia surgery: from Bowditch to laparoscopy. Ann Surg. 2005;241(1):185–93.
32. Weijenborg PW, van Hoeij FB, Smout AJ, Bredenoord AJ. Accuracy of hiatal hernia detection with esophageal high-resolution manometry. Neurogastroenterol Motil. 2015;27(2):293–9.
33. Bredenoord AJ, Hemmink GJ, Smout AJ. Relationship between gastro-oesophageal reflux pattern and severity of mucosal damage. Neurogastroenterol Motil. 2009;21(8):807–12.
34. Herbella FA, Raz DJ, Nipomnick I, Patti MG. Primary versus secondary esophageal motility disorders: diagnosis and implications for treatment. J Lapatoendosc Adv Surg Tech A. 2009;19(2):95–8. 30.
35. Martinucci I, de Bortoli N, Giacchino M, Bodini G, Marabotto E, Marchi S, Savarino V, Savarino E. Esophageal motility abnormalities in gastroesophageal reflux disease. World J Gastrointest Pharmacol Ther. 2014;5(2):86–96.
36. Peters JH, Avisar N. The molecular pathogenesis of Barrett's esophagus: common signaling pathways in embryogenesis metaplasia and neoplasia. J Gastrointest Surg. 2010;14(Suppl 1):S81–7.

37. Theisen J, Peters JH, Fein M, Hughes M, Hagen JA, Demeester SR, Demeester TR, Laird PW. The mutagenic potential of duodenoesophageal reflux. Ann Surg. 2005;241:63–8.
38. Katayama RC, Herbella FAM, Patti MG, Arasaki CH, Oliveira RO, de Grande AC. Laparoscopic sleeve gastrectomy lacks intrasurgeon and intersurgeon agreement in technical key points that may affect gastroesophageal reflux disease after the procedure. Obes Surg. 2024;34(2):542–8. https://doi.org/10.1007/s11695-023-07016-0. Epub 2023 Dec 29.

Medical Therapy for GERD

Jeremy A. Klein and Robert T. Kavitt

Lifestyle Modification

Lifestyle modifications remain first line treatment for gastroesophageal reflux disease (GERD). These modifications limit the pathologic reflux of acidic gastric contents into the esophagus [1, 2]. Recommendations can be grouped into three categories: avoidance of foods that precipitate reflux (caffeine, chocolate, peppermint, alcohol, fatty foods), avoidance of spicy/acidic foods that promote heartburn (citrus, grapefruit, orange, tomatoes), and behaviors that improve lower esophageal sphincter (LES) functioning (smoking cessation, avoidance of recumbent position for 2–3 hours after meals, raising head of bed, sleeping in left lateral decubitus position, and weight loss) [3].

Prior studies found that alcohol, carbonation, tobacco, high-fat foods, peppermint, citrus, and chocolate reduces LES tone and contractility which exacerbates GERD [4]. Therefore, it is physiologically feasible that decreasing exposure to these agents could improve reflux symptoms. The evidence base for many lifestyle modifications is equivocal as controlled studies are difficult to perform. Several randomized controlled trials found head of bed elevation, left-side down sleeping, and weight loss improved GERD symptoms [5–7]. LES tone can also be decreased by hormones such as estrogen and progesterone during pregnancy [8]. Lifestyle modifications, including avoiding triggers, are the foundation for all GERD treatment because it is safe and low risk.

J. A. Klein
Department of Medicine, University of Chicago, Chicago, IL, USA
e-mail: Jeremy.Klein@uchicagomedicine.org

R. T. Kavitt (✉)
Center for Esophageal Diseases, Department of Medicine, Section of Gastroenterology, Hepatology, and Nutrition, University of Chicago, Chicago, IL, USA
e-mail: rkavitt@bsd.uchicago.edu

F. Schlottmann et al. (eds.), *Esophageal Disorders*,
https://doi.org/10.1007/978-3-032-08179-7_3

Postprandial recumbency and raising the head of the bed 6–8 inches uses the protective effect of gravity to improve esophageal acid exposure and promote esophageal healing [5, 9, 10]. Data around the timing of meals prior to bedtime has been conflicting. A small prospective trial showed that participants eating 6 hours prior to supine position (sleeping) had less reflux episodes compared to participants that ate 2 hours prior to bedtime [11]. Thus, it is recommended to avoid eating less than 2 hours before sleeping.

Studies show a dose-dependent relationship between BMI and GERD symptoms [7, 12, 13]. Therefore, weight loss continues to be a recommendation for overweight patients with GERD. Overweight individuals tend to eat more processed fats and consume known dietary triggers of GERD. They also have increased intra-abdominal pressure leading to higher gastroesophageal pressure gradients and increased incidence of hiatal hernias [14]. A Norwegian prospective population-based study of women found lowering BMI by >3.5 kg/m^2 led to less GERD symptoms and augments anti-reflux therapy [7]. Similarly, the 2000 Nurses' Health Study questionnaire found losing >3.5 kg/m^2 was associated with a 40% risk reduction of GERD symptoms [12]. Weight loss can also improve LES functioning and decrease esophageal acid exposure [15]. Even with lifestyle interventions, these modifications alone are not sufficient for the majority of patients with severe or refractory symptoms.

Non-proton Pump Inhibitor-Based Medical Therapy

Non-absorbable Agents

Antacids

Antacids are inorganic salts varying in formulation (chewing gum, chewable, liquids) and potency (greatest to least): calcium carbonate, sodium bicarbonate, magnesium, aluminum salts [16]. Chewing gums offer repetitive esophageal exposure leading to sustained symptom relief and pH control [17]. Unfortunately, antacids do not affect the volume of acid secretion and calcium carbonate formulations are associated with gastric acid-rebound. Along with neutralizing gastric acid, antacids exert a potent effect on increasing esophageal pH [18]. Antacids are likely as effective as H2Rs in healing esophagitis [19].

Limited head-to-head studies exist showing significant symptomatic improvement with antacids compared to placebo or other anti-reflux medications. In general, antacids are well tolerated but can cause adverse effects at higher doses and/or prolonged use. Magnesium compounds can worsen diarrhea, aluminum-based antacids can cause constipation and calcium-based antacids can cause worsened bloating/flatulence. They are short-acting, lasting around 60 minutes per dose [20]. Given the lack of systemic absorption, antacids (aside from magnesium trisilicate and sodium bicarbonate due to side effects) are first line for pregnant patients [21]. For patients with mild GERD symptoms, antacids remain a safe, cheap, on-demand, and fast acting over-the-counter option for temporary heartburn relief.

Alginate

Alginates are natural polysaccharide polymers of variable composition that create a mechanical barrier to reflux. Gastric acid plus alginate precipitates a viscous gel of near-neutral pH. This mechanical barrier acts as a gel raft that pushes the postprandial acid pocket further from the gastro-esophageal junction [22]. These effects reduce reflux for up to 4 hours after dose [23]. In patients with non-erosive GERD, alginates (along with alginate-antacid combination) effectively reduce symptoms compared to placebo [24]. A 2017 meta-analysis showed a trend towards alginates being less effective at symptom reduction compared to H2Ras and PPIs, but this finding was not statistically significant [23]. Additionally, one study found the combination antacid-alginate formulation more effective than antacid alone in controlling postprandial esophageal acid exposure [25]. The main adverse effect is constipation from the aluminum hydroxide. Alginates are likely most effective in patients with postprandial predominant pyrosis and can be used as adjunctive therapy for patients on PPIs [26].

Sucralfate

Sucralfate is an aluminum non-absorbable salt that coats gastric and esophageal mucosa. Use is reserved for pregnant patients as it was found more effective than placebo in controlling GERD symptoms [27]. Sucralfate (along with antacids) are minimally secreted in breast milk and considered safe during lactation [21]. A randomized, double-blind, placebo controlled study at 6 centers in Germany showed superiority of sucralfate compared to placebo for symptomatic management of non-erosive GERD [28]. Current recommendations do not support sucralfate in non-pregnant patients.

Inhibitors of Transient Lower Esophageal Sphincter Relaxations (TLESRs)

For patients on PPI maintenance therapy, GERD symptoms may persist because of continued reflux of gastric contents despite adequate gastric acid suppression. To combat this, agents that inhibit transient lower esophageal sphincter relaxations (TLESRs) have been developed. TLESRs can be inhibited through various pathways, predominately via gamma-aminobutyric acid (GABA) and metabotropic glutamate receptor 5 (mGluR5). TLESRs can also be reduced through lifestyle measures such as sleeping in the left lateral decubitus position [29]. Baclofen (a GABA-B agonist) is one of the few agents that reduce TLESRs and reflux symptoms. A mGluR5 antagonist, Mavoglurant, has been shown to reduce meal-time reflux in a small randomized clinical trial though more research is needed [30].

One RCT of patients with GERD showed that baclofen decreased the number of upright reflex episodes and improved belching/overall symptom score compared to placebo [31]. Additionally, a meta-analysis of 9 randomized controlled trials found that baclofen reduced the average length of reflux episodes, amount of episodes, and the incidence of TLESRs compared to placebo [32]. As Baclofen crosses the blood-brain barrier, dose-related adverse effects such as drowsiness, confusion, and confusion are possible along with nausea/vomiting. Baclofen before meals can be an adjunctive therapy for patients on maintenance PPI with ongoing symptoms.

Anti-secretory Agents

Histamine-2 Receptor Blockers (H2RAs)

H2RAs bind competitively and reversibly to H2 receptors on parietal cells to reduce histamine binding and subsequent gastric acid production. They are offered over-the-counter (Famotidine and Cimetidine) or by prescription (Famotidine, Cimetidine, and Nizatidine) (Table 1). These agents are another common anti-reflux option, often used for patients on PPIs with persistent nocturnal symptoms. Nocturnal acid breakthrough (NAB) occurs in over 70% of patients on PPI therapy [33, 34]. H2RAs last longer compared to antacids but are not as rapid acting (concentrations peak on average 2 hours after dosing).

A meta-analysis of 8 randomized controlled trials found adding H2RA at bedtime decreased the amount of nocturnal reflux episodes [35]. However, studies have found repeated nightly use causes tolerance (tachyphylaxis) to occur in as short as days to weeks [36]. Meta-analysis has shown H2RAs are inferior to PPI alone for symptom relief and treating erosive esophagitis [37]. Another meta-analysis of 13 randomized controlled trials found 80 mg of Famotidine the most effective H2RA for short-term relief [38]. H2RAs are pregnancy category B and are considered safer than PPIs. The main side effects of H2RAs are headache, drowsiness, and fatigue from central antihistamine effects. Prolonged high-dose Cimetidine has been linked to gynecomastia, impotence, and galactorrhea [39] (Table 1).

Table 1 Pharmacokinetics of H2RAs

	Formulation	Dose (mg)	Max dose (mg), CrCl <30 ml/min	Bioavailability (%)	Time to peak (range, hours)	Renal Clearance (%) Oral | IV		Hepatic Clearance (%) Oral | IV		Adverse Effects (in order of incidence)
Famotidine (Pepcid)	Tablet Suspension Intravenous	10, 20, 40 40 mg/5 ml 20	20	40	1–3.5	25–30	65–80	50–80	25–30	Agitation, headache, diarrhea > constipation, dizziness
Cimetidine (Tagamet)	Tablet Solution	200–800 400 mg/6.67 ml	600	80	1–2	40	50–80	60	25–40	Headache, gynecomastia, agitation, dizziness, drowsiness, diarrhea
Nizatidine (Tazac, Axid)	Capsule Solution	150, 300 15 mg/ml	150	70	1–3	57–65	75	22	25	Headache, dizziness, pruritus

Detailed pharmacokinetic data for H2-Receptor antagonists along with common adverse effects. Rare adverse effects <1% not included

Potassium Competitive Acid Blockers (P-CABs)

P-CABs compete with potassium and bind selectively to the proton pump ATPase (alpha subunit). This causes a rapid, dose-dependent, and reversible inhibition of gastric parietal cell acid production [40]. Various P-CABs have been developed since 1980 with the prototype SCH28080 from Schering-Plough Corporation. This compound failed to make it to practice because of hepatotoxicity concerns and non-superiority to PPIs [41]. The first P-CAB, Revaprazan, made it to clinical practice in South Korea and India in 2007 [40]. A recent 2019 phase 3 multi-center randomized controlled clinical trial in South Korea found a novel P-CAB, Tegoprazan (50 or 100 mg daily) non-inferior to esomeprazole 40 mg daily in treating erosive esophagitis [42]. The main benefits of P-CABs compared to PPIs are that P-CABS are more stable in an acidic gastric environment, more concentrated in the parietal cell secretory canaliculi, acts directly on H+/K + -ATPase (compared to PPIs that require transformation to active form), and achieve full effect after the first dose [43]. Vonoprazan effect also appears to be independent of CYP2C19 polymorphism offering a more consistent effect across ethnicities [44].

Due to their potency and long duration of action, P-CABs have an evolving role in refractory GERD. At the time of publication, TAK-438 (Vonoprazan—10 mg or 20 mg daily) is the only P-CAB currently FDA approved for use in GERD and NERD (Table 2). Three others (tegoprazan, fexuprazan and keverprazan) are available in other parts of the world along with ongoing pre-clinical development for linaprazan and zestaprazan [43]. It has already been approved for GERD treatment in Japan (2015) and *Helicobacter Pylori* treatment in the USA (2022). Guidelines from the ACG still recommend bismuth quadruple therapy (PPI, bismuth, metronidazole, and tetracycline) as first-line for eradication of *H. pylori* in treatment-naïve individuals [45]. The AGA subsequently recommended P-CAB-amoxicillin dual therapy over PPIs in eradication regimens for most patients with *Helicobacter pylori* infection given tolerability and lower pill burden [46]. A recent 2022 meta-analysis of 19 studies found Vonoprazan superior to PPI in treating erosive esophagitis, but non-inferior to PPIs in non-erosive esophagitis [47]. Unlike PPIs, P-CABs are not prodrugs, do not require acid activation, and reach maximum plasma concentration in around 2 hours with longer half-life of ~9 hours compared to ~2 hours for most PPIs [48]. Moreover, P-CABs slowly dissociate from the proton pump and maintain mucosal activity for up to 24 hours after administration [49]. The main adverse effects of Vonoprazan is diarrhea and, unlike early P-CABs, no hepatotoxicity was noted [48]. The safety profile at 52 weeks is like lansoprazole [50]. In adults with erosive esophagitis, a non-inferiority randomized trial between PPIs and P-CABs showed higher healing rates at 8 weeks with Vonoprazan 20 mg compared to lansoprazole 30 mg [51]. At 24 weeks, similar rates of healing were seen between Vonoprazan 10 mg and 20 mg with both superior to lansoprazole 15 mg [51]. This effect was more pronounced in patients with more severe LA grade esophagitis C/D [51]. A 2024 systematic review and meta-analysis that included 11 studies and 4108 patients with GERD found P-CABs more effective than PPIs at treating erosive esophagitis (OR: 1.67, 95% CI: 1.24–2.24, $p < 0.01$) [52]. No difference in adverse

Table 2 Pharmacokinetics of PCAB

	Formulation	Dose (mg)	Max dose (mg)with CrCl <30 ml/min	Bioavailability	Half-life (hours)	Time to peak (range, hours)	Hepatic Metabolism Enzyme	Adverse Effects
Vonoprazan (Voquezna)	Tablet	10, 20	Use not recommended	Unknown	7.7	1.5–5.0	CYP3A4	Diarrhea/constipation, nausea/vomit, abdominal pain, rash

Pharmacokinetics of Vonoprazan (novel PCAB) and common adverse effects. Rare adverse effects <1% not included

Table 3 PPI versus P-CAB

	Mechanism of proton pump inhibition	Prodrug; acid required for activation	Concentration in parietal cell compared to plasma	Timing to full effect	Potency	Onset
P-CAB	Reversible	No; does not require acid for activation	100,000-fold	After first dose	↑↑↑↑	Rapid
PPI	Irreversible	Yes; requires acidic environment for activation	1000-fold	Full effects in 2–4 days (requires repeat dosing)	↑↑↑	Slower

Comparison between PPI and P-CABs

events was identified between P-CABs and PPIs. More robust head-to-head comparisons of PPI versus P-CAB therapy is needed to assess maintenance therapy for GERD (Table 3 compares P-CAB to PPI). P-CABs have the potential to augment future anti-reflux care, particularly for patients with erosive disease or PPI-refractory symptoms.

Currently, the practical use of P-CABs is limited largely by cost, insurance coverage, and medication accessibility. For example, Medicare part D does not include coverage of Vonoprazan. More pharmacies are starting to include P-CABs as formulary and the manufacturer offers a co-pay assistance program for commercial insurance.

Proton Pump Inhibitors (PPIs)

Brief Background of PPIs

Proton pump inhibitors (PPIs) potently and irreversibly block the final step of gastric parietal cell acid production. PPIs were developed in the late 1970s, put into practice in the late 1980s, and remain ubiquitous in acid suppression therapy. Omeprazole was taken to human trials in 1982 then launched as Losec in Europe (1988) and as Prilosec in the United States (1990) [53]. Since induction, a 1995 meta-analysis of 30 double-blind prospective trials showed 20 mg of omeprazole daily had greater therapeutic benefit compared to H2RA in symptom resolution, healing erosive esophagitis, duodenal ulcer, gastric ulcers, relapse reduction, maintenance therapy [54, 55].

A 1996 meta-analysis demonstrated PPIs superior to H2RAs, sucralfate, and placebo for heartburn relief and healing of erosive esophagitis [56]. In a 2013 Cochrane review of 34 trials with empiric PPI use, PPIs were deemed more effective than H2RAs in relieving heartburn [57]. As of 2022, there are 6 PPIs (Omeprazole (OTC), Esomeprazole (OTC), Lansoprazole, Dexlansoprazole, Pantoprazole, and Rabeprazole) approved by the FDA for reflux treatment with various formulations: intravenous, enteric-coated, gelatin capsules, coated granules, immediate release, delayed release, multiple-unit pellet system (MUPS), among others [58] (Table 4). Since 2013, PPI use continues to increase as an empiric PPI trial (4 to 8 weeks) remains the recommended initial approach to typical GERD symptoms in patients without alarm symptoms [2].

Pharmacology of PPIs

PPIs covalently bind to the H^+/K^+ ATPase thus inhibiting the 1:1 exchange of intracellular hydrogen for extracellular potassium [59]. PPIs are weak bases that selectively accumulate in stimulated parietal cell canaliculi. This stimulation occurs in response to meals via various secretagogues that induce acid secretion from gastric parietal cells. This acidic environment allows accumulation (1000-fold greater than the concentration of PPI in blood), conversion, and subsequent protonation of the prodrug to the activated cation [59, 60]. As a result, acid secretion can be delayed and is inhibited until replacement pumps are synthesized in a process that can take up to 48 hours [59]. Proton pump recovery is independent of the PPI dose. It is recommended to take PPIs at least 30 minutes prior to meals to exert their antacid effect on activated proton pumps. If PPIs are combined with other anti-secretory or antacid agents then the PPI effect will be dampened as gastric acid secretion relies on negative feedback [61].

In a prolonged fasted state, many proton pumps are inactive, with greater potential for activation and acid release upon stimulus exposure. Therefore, PPIs are more effective in this setting when a larger number of proton pumps are activated [62]. Not all parietal cells or proton pumps are simultaneously activated due to this dynamic process. As a result of this and the PPI plasma half-life of ~90 minutes, orally dosed PPIs inhibit around 70% of proton pumps [59] (Table 4). Yet, because of the irreversible binding, PPIs exert an inhibitory effect on acid secretion for up to 48 hours [59]. On once daily PPI dosing, acid inhibition takes about 2–3 days to achieve steady state [59]. Oral bioavailability is high, on average about 85%, for all PPIs [58].

PPIs are protein-bound and mainly metabolized via hepatic CYP2C19 and 3A4 enzymes with CYP activity varying between individual phenotypes. Some Europeans and North Americans are genetically rapid metabolizers, which can explain a lack of response [58]. Others are poor metabolizers that lack CYP2C19 (3% of Caucasians and 15%–20% of Asians) leading to prolonged half-life and systemic drug exposure [59].

Omeprazole

Omeprazole was developed in the 1970s and approved by the FDA in 1989. Omeprazole is offered over-the-counter (20 mg) and as intravenous, capsules, tablets, immediate release (IR), delayed-release, multiple-unit pellet system (MUPS), and oral suspension. It has lower bioavailability at ~35%, the fastest onset (0.5–3.5 hours), and the shortest half-life (0.5–1 hour) compared to other PPIs [58]. Omeprazole-IR/sodium bicarbonate suspension is non-enteric coated, rapid acting, and superior to pantoprazole delayed-release, esomeprazole, and lansoprazole in reducing nocturnal acid breakthrough symptoms [63, 64]. This is likely due to

Table 4 PPI pharmacodynamics

	Brand Name	Over the counter?	Formulation (IV, DR, capsule, suspension, ODT)	Dose (mg)	Bioavailability (~%)	Half-life (hours)	Time to peak (range, hours)	Hepatic Metabolism Enzyme	Adverse Effects (in order of incidence)
Omeprazole	Prilosec Zegerid (sodium bicarbonate)	Yes	Tablet-DR Capsule-DR Suspension Packet	20 10, 20, 40 10, 20 2.5–10	30–40	0.5–1.2	0.5–3.5	CYP2C19	Headache, abdominal pain, diarrhea, nausea, dizziness, rash, upper respiratory infection
Pantoprazole	Protonix	No	Tablet-DR Packet Intravenous	20, 40 40 40	77	0.8–2.0	2–3	CYP2C19, CYP3A4	[a]Headache, diarrhea, upper respiratory tract infection, rash, hypersensitivity reaction, myalgia
Esomeprazole	Nexium	Yes	Tablet-DR Packet Capsule-DR Intravenous	20 2.5–40 20, 40 20, 40	64–90	1.0–1.5	1.5	CYP2C19	Headache, abdominal pain, diarrhea, constipation, dizziness
Lansoprazole	Prevacid	Yes	Capsule-DR Suspension Dissolvable	15, 30	80–85	0.9–2.1	1.7	CYP2C19	Abdominal pain, diarrhea, headache, constipation, dizziness
Dexlansoprazole	Dexilant	No	Capsules-DR	30, 60	—	1–2	1–2, 4–5	CYP2C19, CYP3A4	Headache, diarrhea, upper respiratory tract infection
Rabeprazole	Aciphex	No	Sprinkle Tablets-DR	5, 10 20	52	1–2	2–5	CYP2C19	Abdominal pain, diarrhea, vomiting, headache, pharyngitis

Detailed table of Proton Pump Inhibitors, pharmacodynamics, formulations, and common adverse effects (ordered by incidence)
[a]Higher incidence with IV versus oral formulations. Rare adverse effects <1% not included

sodium bicarbonate acting as a buffer to rapidly neutralize gastric acid, thus activating more proton pumps and protecting the uncoated tablet [65]. However, clinical significance remains at question after a 2015 phase 3 clinical trial did not find immediate-release omeprazole superior to delayed-release in self-reported symptom improvement [66]. Further studies are needed to evaluate immediate-release and the correlation between intragastric pH, heartburn relief, and quality of life. Omeprazole is the only PPI that is safety class C during pregnancy because of increased fetal mortality in animal models [21].

Esomeprazole

Esomeprazole is an isomer of omeprazole, approved by the FDA in 2001 for the treatment of GERD and erosive esophagitis. It is available in 20 mg or 40 mg, intravenous, liquid, immediate-release, delayed-release, and multiple-unit pellet system (MUPS) formulations. The oral bioavailability after 40 mg daily increased with repeated doses up to 90% after day 5 with a half-life of ~1.5 hours [67]. A 2006 meta-analysis of 10 studies reported a 5% relative increase in erosive esophagitis healing probability at 8 weeks with esomeprazole compared to pantoprazole, lansoprazole, and omeprazole (number-needed-to-treat of 25) [68]. Other studies have found esomeprazole 40 mg more effective at controlling intragastric pH (mean percentage of time with pH >4 over 24 hours) compared to omeprazole 40 mg, pantoprazole 40 mg, rabeprazole 20 mg, or lansoprazole 30 mg once daily [69–71]. When divided into two doses per day, even better intragastric pH control was achieved with esomeprazole 40 mg twice daily compared to other PPIs [72]. Despite numerous meta-analyses reporting greater efficacy of esomeprazole, the clinical significance of these differences is to be seen [73].

Pantoprazole

Pantoprazole was first approved in Germany in 1994 and then in 2000 by the FDA for treatment of erosive esophagitis [74]. At the time, it was the first PPI available in intravenous and oral formulations (delayed-release, oral suspension). In 2001, the FDA approved IV Pantoprazole 40 mg once daily for 7–10 days in patients with GERD and a history of erosive esophagitis unable to tolerate oral medication [74]. Unlike other PPIs, serum concentration is not dose-dependent [75]. Pantoprazole binds to cysteine 822 residues which make it more stoichiometrically challenging for reducing agents (such as glutathione) to reverse pantoprazole activity. Thus, pantoprazole reversal relies more heavily on de novo pump synthesis [76].

In a study of 603 patients with erosive esophagitis, results showed pantoprazole 40 mg/day offered early esophagitis healing and had the highest healing rates at 4 and 8 weeks compared to other pantoprazole doses [77]. However, pantoprazole offered no difference in endoscopic healing rates at 4 or 8 weeks compared to omeprazole 20 mg/day or lansoprazole 30 mg/day [78]. Other studies comparing pantoprazole 40 mg/day to esomeprazole 40 mg/day found patients taking pantoprazole had less symptomatic episodes at one week [79] and faster first time nocturnal symptom relief [80]. With robust data in over 100 clinical trials, pantoprazole is an established safe, well-tolerated, and effective PPI.

Lansoprazole

Lansoprazole (LAN) comes in delayed release oral disintegrating tablet and a novel fast disintegrated tablet (LFDT) that is easily swallowed with or without water [60, 81]. The fast-disintegrating tablet is easily mixed into drinks/food; this improves patient convenience and tolerability for older individuals, children, patients with dysphagia, nothing-per-oral (NPO) status, and those with nasogastric tubes. Several studies suggest that compared to omeprazole, lansoprazole offers more effective acid control with a quicker onset of action (~1.5 hours) [82]. Along with above formulations, lansoprazole comes in intravenous, liquid suspension, and 15 mg or 30 mg capsules [58]. Compared to other PPIs, lansoprazole has the highest oral bioavailability around 80% and a longer half-life of ~1.6 hours [58].

Dexlansoprazole

Dexlansoprazole is available in 30 mg and 60 mg delayed release capsules and oral disintegrating tablet. The delayed release formulation offers longer half-life than other PPI agents [83]. The granule composition has different pH dissolution properties that allows for around 25% of drug release into the proximal duodenum and the remaining portion in small bowel. This prolongs plasma concentration, reaching peak ~2 hours and then again at 5 hours after administration [83]. Unlike other PPIs, dexlansoprazole reaches higher plasma concentration when administered 30 minutes after a meal. For those unable to adhere to meal-time restrictions, dexlansoprazole takes the onus off patients [84]. A meta-analysis of 11 randomized trials found 4 weeks of dexlansoprazole 30 mg is more efficacious compared to esomeprazole (40 mg; RR: 2.17, 95% CI: 1.39–3.38) in controlling GERD symptoms [85].

Rabeprazole

Rabeprazole, approved in 2002, is available in 10 mg, 20 mg, delayed and extended-release 50 mg tablets. It has a slower onset than other PPI at 2–5 hours with a half-life of 1–2 hours [58]. The extended release formulation is gradually absorbed throughout the small intestine and colon to improve serum half-life [58]. One Canadian study of 248 healthy volunteers found rabeprazole-DR 20 mg had superior nocturnal acid suppression compared to esomeprazole 40 mg [86]. A different study, in patients with erosive esophagitis, found Rabeprazole-ER was not superior to esomeprazole in improving heartburn symptoms or esophageal healing [87]. Compared to other PPIs, Rabeprazole 20 mg is the most potent PPI available and can be used second line in patients with persistent symptoms after an initial PPI trial.

Drug Interactions

PPIs are highly protein-bound and metabolized largely via the CYP2C19 pathway (though pantoprazole and dexlansoprazole also have CYP3A4 metabolism) [58]. Individuals metabolize PPIs at different rates due to genetic variations in the CYP pathway [60]. Omeprazole and esomeprazole have the highest percentage of CYP2C19 metabolism conferring the greatest drug-drug interaction risk [58]. Less drug-drug interactions are seen with lansoprazole, pantoprazole, dexlansoprazole, and rabeprazole due to the affinity for CYP3A4 degradation [58]. Along with effects on cytochrome degradation, PPIs can affect the solubility/bioavailability of medications that rely on a more acidic gastric environment [88].

Observational research over the past 15 years has focused on the potential interaction between clopidogrel and PPIs given clopidogrel requires CYP2C19 activation [89]. This concern is greatest with CYP2C19-dependent PPIs. Despite the proposed risk of decreased clopidogrel activation, multiple randomized trials have not shown an increased risk of adverse cardiovascular events with clopidogrel and PPI co-ingestion [90]. Moreover, separating administration by 12–20 hours (~3 clopidogrel half-lives) may prevent competitive CYP inhibition and limit a clinically significant interaction [91, 92]. Along with clopidogrel, concomitant administration of PPI with various medications (such as mycophenolate, levothyroxine, digoxin, etc.) can increase the risk for adverse effect [89].

Long-Term PPI Therapy

Safety concerns of prolonged PPI therapy have been well documented. Especially in an era of technology, information accessibility, and over-the-counter medications, it is important that patients have an accurate understanding of PPI risks and benefits. Many adverse events linked to PPIs are associations made from epidemiologic studies. These putative adverse effects include pneumonia, acute kidney injury, gastrointestinal infections, nutritional deficiencies, osteoporosis, dementia, and others. Many reported effects lack evidence of causality plus limitations from inherent biases and confounding variables. A 2019 randomized placebo-controlled prospective clinical trial with 17,598 patients and about 3 years of follow-up did not find any statistically significant adverse effects associated with pantoprazole use [93]. This is the largest prospective trial assessing adverse effects of PPI use. As a drug class, PPIs are overall well-tolerated with a few non-specific side effects. These include but are not limited to headaches, dizziness, rash, nausea, vomiting, abdominal pain, constipation, diarrhea [94]. When medication is halted, these side effects dissipate.

PPI use has been linked to community (CAP) and hospital acquired pneumonia (HAP), hypothesized due to micro-aspiration of gastric contents. Concern for this link grew in 2004 after JAMA published a study reporting a positive dose-response and an adjusted relative risk of 1.89 for patients on PPI versus those that stopped [95]. This association was further assessed in a systematic review of 26 studies that found outpatient PPI use conferred a 1.5-fold increased risk of CAP [96]. Another large pharmacoepidemiologic cohort study found PPIs linked to a 30% increased odds of HAP [97]. Some studies suggest this risk is greatest within 30 days of starting PPI therapy [96, 98], decreasing the likelihood that PPIs could directly cause pneumonia in such a time frame. Other studies suggest this association is limited by comorbid conditions, temporal feasibility, and protopathic bias where early symptoms of pneumonia were falsely attributed to GERD and treated with PPIs [99–101].

Along with pneumonia, PPIs and its associated hypochlorhydria (gastric acid deficiency) has been linked to gastrointestinal infections like small intestinal bacterial overgrowth (SIBO) and *Clostridium difficile* infection (CDI). Prior studies evaluating SIBO risk from PPI use have been conflicting with a 2018 meta-analysis conferring moderate risk (pooled OR 1.71) [102]. This relative risk increases eightfold when SIBO is diagnosed with duodenal aspirates [103]. However, objective findings of SIBO do not always correlate with symptomatic and clinically relevant infection.

For CDI, *C. difficile* spores are not sensitive to gastric acid. Therefore, it is hypothesized that the lack of gastric acid allows for the survival of the toxin-forming vegetative state [101]. Another explanation is the loss of microbial diversity in the colon after PPI use leading to diminished endogenous barriers to *C. difficile* infection [104–107]. A meta-analysis of 56 studies found PPI use significantly associated with increased risk of CDI (including when stratifying for study type), though these studies are limited again by bias from observational/retrospective design [108]. Other studies have found that concurrent PPI and *C. difficile* treatment does not increase risk of CDI recurrence [107].

In 2019, results were released from the COMPASS randomized controlled trial that added more real-word context. This study assessed cardiovascular outcomes over 3 years for patients on various doses of rivaroxaban with or without aspirin. In addition, the study had PPI-related arms containing 17,598 patients at 580 centers. Over the 3-year study, adverse effects were reported with a very slight increased risk of enteric infections (1.33; 95% confidence interval, 1.01–1.75) [93]. More prospective studies or randomized clinical trials are needed to further contextualize the severity and clinical significance of the many reported adverse effects of PPIs.

There is also consideration regarding micronutrient malabsorption due to altered gastric microbiome and the less acidic environment. Of particular concern is the absorption of calcium, B12, magnesium, and iron. Gastric acid facilitates ionized calcium release from calcium salts [106], though PPIs have less effect on calcium contained in dairy and water-soluble calcium salts [109]. Studies have yet to show strong evidence that chronic PPI exposure causes B12 deficiency, though a case-control study from 2013 found an increased odds risk for B12 deficiency in patients that had been prescribed a PPI [110]. Like B12, gastric acid is needed for optimal iron reduction and absorption. A case-control study found PPI use >2 years and higher dose were associated with increased risk of iron deficiency anemia [111]. Another case-control study found a positive dose-response and time-response relationship to chronic PPI use >1 year and risk of iron deficiency [112]. Gastric acid is also important for the absorption of non-heme iron, which requires an acidic environment to facilitate reduction of ferric iron to ferrous state [113]. More prospective research is needed to determine if PPIs cause clinically significant iron deficiency [111].

Alterations in serum magnesium is another adverse effect of active research despite magnesium absorption occurring passively throughout the small intestine independent of gastric acid. The mechanism is not fully elucidated and current meta-analyses literature is not conclusive as prior study populations were heterogenous [114]. Yet, some studies found serum magnesium levels recovered quickly after PPI discontinuation (an effect not seen with H2-blockers) [115]. Patients on PPIs are also resistant to magnesium supplementation [115]. These findings led to a 2011 FDA safety announcement about the potential link between PPI exposure >1 year and hypomagnesemia. Still, the 2022 ACG Clinical Guidelines do not recommend routine monitoring or supplementation of magnesium, calcium, B12, or iron for patients on PPI therapy [4].

PPI use can feasibly impact bone health from altered calcium absorption, direct inhibition of osteoclast activity, and gastrin-mediated parathyroid hyperplasia [116]. Some observational studies including two large meta-analysis have found a modest association between PPI use and hip or vertebral fracture risk [117–119]. However, like other PPI side effects, the clinical relevance and causal relationship of PPI use and bone health remains controversial, especially given that fracture risk is a complex and confounded composite outcome [120, 121]. In 2010 the FDA announced a safety warning for the possible link between long-term PPI use and hip, wrist, and spine fracture risk. This caution statement was revised in 2011 to exclude fracture risk associated with short term OTC PPI use due to lower doses and less exposure time. More recent meta-analysis in 2018, 2020 and 2022 report conflicting findings between PPI and bone mineral density. While fracture incidence trended higher in PPI users, there has not been convincing evidence linking PPI to decreased bone mineral density [119, 122, 123]. The 2022 ACG Clinical Guidelines do not recommend additional bone mineral density screening for patients on PPIs [4].

Multiple meta-analyses and retrospective population-based studies have linked PPIs to acute kidney injury (AKI), acute interstitial nephritis (AIN), risk of chronic kidney disease (CKD), CKD progression, and end-stage renal disease (ESRD) [124–126]. A nested population based, case-control study in New Zealand found AIN occurred at a higher rate in current PPI users compared to past PPI users (patients not on PPI >90 days prior to AIN diagnosis) [125]. Another large retrospective cohort study found an association between PPI exposure and AKI incidence (adjusted odds ratio 4.35, 3.14–6.04, $p < 0.0001$) [126]. Similar studies have found an increased incidence of CKD in patients exposed to PPI therapy [126]. CKD risk also increases with prolonged exposure [124, 127] and higher PPI doses [128]. A retrospective cohort analysis of ~125,000 PPI user and found over 50% of patients had PPI-associated chronic renal injury irrespective of predisposing AKI [129]. This, along with other studies, points toward more variable and indolent kidney injury than typical immune-mediated drug nephrotoxicity [125, 130]. Thus, preceding AKI cannot be reliable used as an indicator of PPI toxicity and routine monitoring of kidney function is not standard of care [4]. However, patients with other risk factors and comorbidities may warrant closer creatinine monitoring and necessity of PPI therapy addressed.

Lastly, data suggests that PPI use may exacerbate development of dementia in elderly patients [131]. Mouse models have shown PPIs can inhibit V-type ATPases in microglial cells leading to less β-amyloid degradation and subsequent amyloid-β

(Aβ) protein deposition [132]. However, studies have been conflicting [133, 134] and a recent 2020 meta-analysis did not show a significant relative risk of PPI use and dementia [123]. Especially in older patients who are subject to polypharmacy, confounding comorbidities, and dementia development, it is challenging to draw conclusions from PPI exposure and dementia progression/risk [109].

Approach to Pharmacologic Therapy

For patients with typical mild reflux symptoms >2 episodes per week without erosive esophagitis or red flag alarm features (dysphagia, odynophagia, weight loss, recurrent vomiting), a step-up approach can be utilized. In this approach, treatment may start with antacids and H2RAs with subsequent dose adjustments in 4 weeks until symptoms are controlled. If symptoms persist, patients should trial daily PPI therapy for 4–8 weeks. If symptoms resolve, it is reasonable to consider PPI on-demand therapy with as needed antacids/H2RA. On the other hand, if symptoms persist then it is important to ensure patients are taking their PPI 30 minutes prior to meals. If medication adherence is confirmed, then patients may switch to a more potent PPI and/or escalate to twice daily dosing (discussed below).

For patients with erosive disease or frequent severe reflux symptoms, a step-down strategy can be employed. These patients may benefit from daily PPI for 8 weeks instead of 4 weeks [135]. If symptoms resolve, then stepping down to H2RAs for maintenance is a feasible approach. If symptoms persist after 8 weeks of PPI therapy, dosing frequency is increased to twice daily [136]. Those that do not respond to twice daily PPI after 12 weeks are deemed to have refractory disease, which can occur in up to 30% of patients with GERD [137]. One clinical trial of patients with mild esophagitis on esomeprazole 40 mg found prolonging therapy from 4 to 8 weeks reduced symptom relapse [135]. Current recommendations are to continue maintenance PPI therapy while exploring other diagnostics and procedural options [4]. This includes an endoscopy off PPI for at least 2 weeks to evaluate for erosive disease and exclude Eosinophilic Esophagitis with biopsies. These patients are also appropriate for pH testing, esophageal manometry, and consideration for pH-impedance to further understand their GERD phenotype.

Many studies and clinical trials have sought to discover how to select the optimal PPI and dosing. PPI potency and efficacy is often assessed using time with gastric pH > 4 as an objective marker. PPI and gastric pH have a linear dose-response with a ceiling effect seen at 70 mg of omeprazole and with three-times daily dosing [138]. In addition, esomeprazole 20 mg and omeprazole 20 mg had similar time of gastric pH > 4 [139]. As a class, PPIs maintained gastric pH > 4 for 15–21 hours per day as compared to 8 hours daily with H2RAs [56]. The World Health Organization proposed that omeprazole 20 mg is equivalent to rabeprazole 20 mg, esomeprazole 30 mg, lansoprazole 30 mg, dexlansoprazole 30 mg, and pantoprazole 40 mg [138]. Vonoprazan 10 mg daily is more potent and equivalent to 60 mg of omeprazole

[138]. Despite omeprazole doses greater than 20 mg per day offering superior acid control and esophagitis healing, it remains uncertain whether this translates to any symptomatic/clinical benefit [140].

For some patients with incomplete responses, switching to another PPI is a feasible approach given the variation of intragastric pH control [58]. A double-blind, randomized study found that for patients with persistent heartburn on lansoprazole 30 mg, increasing to twice daily lansoprazole was as effective as switching to esomeprazole 40 mg [141]. Yet, almost 10% of patients remain symptomatic on twice daily PPI [142]. Those with persistent symptoms unresponsive to initial PPI trial could be genetically rapid drug metabolizers. These patients may benefit from switching to PPIs with limited CYP2C19 metabolism, such as rabeprazole or pantoprazole (lowest cytochrome induction or inhibition amongst benzimidoles) [58]. A randomized control trial of patients on daily PPI showed 20% had symptomatic improvement when increasing to twice-daily PPI or switching PPI [143].

For those patients with ongoing refractory reflux, severe erosive esophagitis LA grade C or D, or recurrent nocturnal symptoms, it is reasonable to consider a mechanistic switch to a P-CAB such as Vonoprazan. P-CABs do not require pre-meal dosing and offers acid control via a different mechanism than PPIs.

Since reflux symptoms are so prevalent, PPIs continue to be amongst the most prescribed medications in many countries [144]. With more attention and research into PPI side effects, many primary care providers and gastroenterologists are reassessing PPI prescribing patterns. As with many medications, timing for dose adjustment or therapy discontinuation is patient specific. Studies have demonstrated lower healthcare costs, improved symptom relief, and unchanged quality of life with full-dose PPI step-down approach compared to H2RA and low-dose PPI step-up strategies [145]. For patients with mild symptoms, one study found omeprazole 10 mg had similar symptomatic remission at 1 year compared to omeprazole 20 mg (77% vs. 83% respectively) [146]. Another multi-center study reported 80% success rate of step-down from omeprazole 20 mg to omeprazole 10 mg [147].

More studies need to be done to assess the clinical significance of PPI discontinuation and subsequent rebound acid hypersecretion. Current evidence points towards tapering patients who have been on PPI therapy for greater than 6 months. For patients with mild to moderate GERD, decreasing maintenance PPI dose offered less symptom relapse compared to "on-demand" PPI or class switch to H2RA [144].

References

1. Kahrilas PJ, Shaheen NJ, Vaezi MF, Institute AGA, Committee CPaQM. American Gastroenterological Association Institute technical review on the management of gastroesophageal reflux disease. Gastroenterology. 2008;135(4):1392–413., 1413.e1–5. https://doi.org/10.1053/j.gastro.2008.08.044.
2. Katz PO, Gerson LB, Vela MF. Guidelines for the diagnosis and management of gastroesophageal reflux disease. Am J Gastroenterol. 2013;108(3):308–28; quiz 329. https://doi.org/10.1038/ajg.2012.444.

3. Kaltenbach T, Crockett S, Gerson LB. Are lifestyle measures effective in patients with gastroesophageal reflux disease? An evidence-based approach. Arch Intern Med. 2006;166(9):965–71. https://doi.org/10.1001/archinte.166.9.965.
4. Katz PO, Dunbar KB, Schnoll-Sussman FH, Greer KB, Yadlapati R, Spechler SJ. ACG clinical guideline for the diagnosis and management of gastroesophageal reflux disease. Am J Gastroenterol. 2022;117(1):27–56. https://doi.org/10.14309/ajg.0000000000001538.
5. Pollmann H, Zillessen E, Pohl J, et al. Effect of elevated head position in bed in therapy of gastroesophageal reflux. Z Gastroenterol. 1996;34(Suppl 2):93–9.
6. Khoury RM, Camacho-Lobato L, Katz PO, Mohiuddin MA, Castell DO. Influence of spontaneous sleep positions on nighttime recumbent reflux in patients with gastroesophageal reflux disease. Am J Gastroenterol. 1999;94(8):2069–73. https://doi.org/10.1111/j.1572-0241.1999.01279.x.
7. Ness-Jensen E, Lindam A, Lagergren J, Hveem K. Weight loss and reduction in gastroesophageal reflux. A prospective population-based cohort study: the HUNT study. Am J Gastroenterol. 2013;108(3):376–82. https://doi.org/10.1038/ajg.2012.466.
8. Richter JE. Gastroesophageal reflux disease during pregnancy. Gastroenterol Clin N Am. 2003;32(1):235–61.
9. Hamilton JW, Boisen RJ, Yamamoto DT, Wagner JL, Reichelderfer M. Sleeping on a wedge diminishes exposure of the esophagus to refluxed acid. Dig Dis Sci. 1988;33(5):518–22.
10. Harvey RF, Gordon PC, Hadley N, et al. Effects of sleeping with the bed-head raised and of ranitidine in patients with severe peptic oesophagitis. Lancet. 1987;2(8569):1200–3.
11. Piesman M, Hwang I, Maydonovitch C, Wong RK. Nocturnal reflux episodes following the administration of a standardized meal. Does timing matter? Am J Gastroenterol. 2007;102(10):2128–34. https://doi.org/10.1111/j.1572-0241.2007.01348.x.
12. Jacobson BC, Somers SC, Fuchs CS, Kelly CP, Camargo CA. Body-mass index and symptoms of gastroesophageal reflux in women. N Engl J Med. 2006;354(22):2340–8. https://doi.org/10.1056/NEJMoa054391.
13. Hampel H, Abraham NS, El-Serag HB. Meta-analysis: obesity and the risk for gastroesophageal reflux disease and its complications. Ann Intern Med. 2005;143(3):199–211.
14. Fraser-Moodie CA, Norton B, Gornall C, Magnago S, Weale AR, Holmes GK. Weight loss has an independent beneficial effect on symptoms of gastro-oesophageal reflux in patients who are overweight. Scand J Gastroenterol. 1999;34(4):337–40.
15. Mathus-Vliegen EM, Tygat GN. Gastro-oesophageal reflux in obese subjects: influence of overweight, weight loss and chronic gastric balloon distension. Scand J Gastroenterol. 2002;37(11):1246–52.
16. Maton PN, Burton ME. Antacids revisited - a review of their clinical pharmacology and recommended therapeutic use. Drugs. 1999;57(6):855–70. https://doi.org/10.2165/00003495-199957060-00003.
17. Collings KL, Rodriguez-Stanley S, Proskin HM, Robinson M, Miner PB. Clinical effectiveness of a new antacid chewing gum on heartburn and oesophageal pH control. Aliment Pharmacol Ther. 2002;16(12):2029–35. https://doi.org/10.1046/j.0269-2813.2002.01380.x.
18. Decktor DL, Robinson M, Maton PN, Lanza FL, Gottlieb S. Effects of aluminum/magnesium hydroxide and calcium carbonate on esophageal and gastric pH in subjects with heartburn. Am J Ther. 1995;2(8):546–52.
19. Graham DY, Patterson DJ. Double-blind comparison of liquid antacid and placebo in the treatment of symptomatic reflux esophagitis. Dig Dis Sci. 1983;28(6):559–63. https://doi.org/10.1007/BF01308159.
20. Garg V, Narang P, Taneja R. Antacids revisited: review on contemporary facts and relevance for self-management. J Int Med Res. 2022;50(3):3000605221086457. https://doi.org/10.1177/03000605221086457.
21. Richter JE. Review article: the management of heartburn in pregnancy. Aliment Pharmacol Ther. 2005;22(9):749–57. https://doi.org/10.1111/j.1365-2036.2005.02654.x.
22. Kwiatek MA, Roman S, Fareeduddin A, Pandolfino JE, Kahrilas PJ. An alginate-antacid formulation (Gaviscon double action liquid) can eliminate or displace the postprandial 'acid

pocket' in symptomatic GERD patients. Aliment Pharmacol Ther. 2011;34(1):59–66. https://doi.org/10.1111/j.1365-2036.2011.04678.x.
23. Leiman DA, Riff BP, Morgan S, et al. Alginate therapy is effective treatment for GERD symptoms: a systematic review and meta-analysis. Dis Esophagus. 2017;30(5):1–9. https://doi.org/10.1093/dote/dow020.
24. Wilkinson J, Wade A, Thomas SJ, Jenner B, Hodgkinson V, Coyle C. Randomized clinical trial: a double-blind, placebo-controlled study to assess the clinical efficacy and safety of alginate-antacid (Gaviscon double action) chewable tablets in patients with gastro-oesophageal reflux disease. Eur J Gastroenterol Hepatol. 2019;31(1):86–93. https://doi.org/10.1097/MEG.0000000000001258.
25. De Ruigh A, Roman S, Chen J, Pandolfino JE, Kahrilas PJ. Gaviscon double action liquid (antacid & alginate) is more effective than antacid in controlling post-prandial oesophageal acid exposure in GERD patients: a double-blind crossover study. Aliment Pharmacol Ther. 2014;40(5):531–7. https://doi.org/10.1111/apt.12857.
26. Manabe N, Haruma K, Ito M, et al. Efficacy of adding sodium alginate to omeprazole in patients with nonerosive reflux disease: a randomized clinical trial. Dis Esophagus. 2012;25(5):373–80. https://doi.org/10.1111/j.1442-2050.2011.01276.x.
27. Phupong V, Hanprasertpong T. Interventions for heartburn in pregnancy. Cochrane Database Syst Rev. 2015;9:CD011379. https://doi.org/10.1002/14651858.CD011379.pub2.
28. Simon B, Ravelli GP, Goffin H. Sucralfate gel versus placebo in patients with non-erosive gastro-oesophageal reflux disease. Aliment Pharmacol Ther. 1996;10(3):441–6. https://doi.org/10.1111/j.0953-0673.1996.00441.x.
29. Loots C, Smits M, Omari T, Bennink R, Benninga M, van Wijk M. Effect of lateral positioning on gastroesophageal reflux (GER) and underlying mechanisms in GER disease (GERD) patients and healthy controls. Neurogastroenterol Motil. 2013;25(3):222–9., e161-2. https://doi.org/10.1111/nmo.12042.
30. Rouzade-Dominguez ML, Pezous N, David OJ, et al. The selective metabotropic glutamate receptor 5 antagonist mavoglurant (AFQ056) reduces the incidence of reflux episodes in dogs and patients with moderate to severe gastroesophageal reflux disease. Neurogastroenterol Motil. 2017;29(8) https://doi.org/10.1111/nmo.13058.
31. Cossentino MJ, Mann K, Armbruster SP, Lake JM, Maydonovitch C, Wong RK. Randomised clinical trial: the effect of baclofen in patients with gastro-oesophageal reflux–a randomised prospective study. Aliment Pharmacol Ther. 2012;35(9):1036–44. https://doi.org/10.1111/j.1365-2036.2012.05068.x.
32. Li S, Shi S, Chen F, Lin J. The effects of baclofen for the treatment of gastroesophageal reflux disease: a meta-analysis of randomized controlled trials. Gastroenterol Res Pract. 2014;2014:307805. https://doi.org/10.1155/2014/307805.
33. Peghini PL, Katz PO, Castell DO. Ranitidine controls nocturnal gastric acid breakthrough on omeprazole: a controlled study in normal subjects. Gastroenterology. 1998;115(6):1335–9. https://doi.org/10.1016/s0016-5085(98)70010-1.
34. Tutuian R, Katz PO, Castell DO. Nocturnal acid breakthrough: pH, drugs and bugs. Eur J Gastroenterol Hepatol. 2004;16(5):441–3.
35. Wang Y, Pan T, Wang Q, Guo Z. Additional bedtime H2-receptor antagonist for the control of nocturnal gastric acid breakthrough. Cochrane Database Syst Rev. 2009;4:CD004275. https://doi.org/10.1002/14651858.CD004275.pub3.
36. McRorie JW, Kirby JA, Miner PB. Histamine2-receptor antagonists: rapid development of tachyphylaxis with repeat dosing. World J Gastrointest Pharmacol Ther. 2014;5(2):57–62. https://doi.org/10.4292/wjgpt.v5.i2.57.
37. Wang WH, Huang JQ, Zheng GF, et al. Head-to-head comparison of H2-receptor antagonists and proton pump inhibitors in the treatment of erosive esophagitis: a meta-analysis. World J Gastroenterol. 2005;11(26):4067–77.
38. Zhao F, Wang S, Liu L, Wang Y. Comparative effectiveness of histamine-2 receptor antagonists as short-term therapy for gastro-esophageal reflux disease: a network meta-analysis. Int J Clin Pharmacol Ther. 2016;54(10):761–70. https://doi.org/10.5414/CP202564.

39. García Rodríguez LA, Jick H. Risk of gynaecomastia associated with cimetidine, omeprazole, and other antiulcer drugs. BMJ. 1994;308(6927):503–6. https://doi.org/10.1136/bmj.308.6927.503.
40. Rawla P, Sunkara T, Ofosu A, Gaduputi V. Potassium-competitive acid blockers – are they the next generation of proton pump inhibitors? World J Gastrointest Pharmacol Ther. 2018;9(7):63–8. https://doi.org/10.4292/wjgpt.v9.i7.63.
41. Oshima T, Miwa H. Potent potassium-competitive acid blockers: a new era for the treatment of acid-related diseases. J Neurogastroenterol Motil. 2018;24(3):334–44. https://doi.org/10.5056/jnm18029.
42. Lee KJ, Son BK, Kim GH, et al. Randomised phase 3 trial: tegoprazan, a novel potassium-competitive acid blocker, vs. esomeprazole in patients with erosive oesophagitis. Aliment Pharmacol Ther. 2019;49(7):864–72. https://doi.org/10.1111/apt.15185.
43. Scarpignato C, Hunt RH. Potassium-competitive acid blockers: current clinical use and future developments. Curr Gastroenterol Rep. 2024;26(11):273–93. https://doi.org/10.1007/s11894-024-00939-3.
44. Scarpignato C, Hunt RH. The potential role of potassium-competitive acid blockers in the treatment of gastroesophageal reflux disease. Curr Opin Gastroenterol. 2019;35(4):344–55. https://doi.org/10.1097/MOG.0000000000000543.
45. Chey WD, Howden CW, Moss SF, et al. ACG clinical guideline: treatment of helicobacter pylori infection. Am J Gastroenterol. 2024;119(9):1730–53. https://doi.org/10.14309/ajg.0000000000002968.
46. Patel A, Laine L, Moayyedi P, Wu J. AGA clinical practice update on integrating potassium-competitive acid blockers into clinical practice: expert review. Gastroenterology. 2024;167(6):1228–38. https://doi.org/10.1053/j.gastro.2024.06.038.
47. Simadibrata DM, Syam AF, Lee YY. A comparison of efficacy and safety of potassium-competitive acid blocker and proton pump inhibitor in gastric acid-related diseases: a systematic review and meta-analysis. J Gastroenterol Hepatol. 2022;37(12):2217–28. https://doi.org/10.1111/jgh.16017.
48. Sugano K. Vonoprazan fumarate, a novel potassium-competitive acid blocker, in the management of gastroesophageal reflux disease: safety and clinical evidence to date. Ther Adv Gastroenterol. 2018;11:1756283X17745776. https://doi.org/10.1177/1756283X17745776.
49. Leowattana W, Leowattana T. Potassium-competitive acid blockers and gastroesophageal reflux disease. World J Gastroenterol. 2022;28(28):3608–19. https://doi.org/10.3748/wjg.v28.i28.3608.
50. Jenkins H, Sakurai Y, Nishimura A, et al. Randomised clinical trial: safety, tolerability, pharmacokinetics and pharmacodynamics of repeated doses of TAK-438 (vonoprazan), a novel potassium-competitive acid blocker, in healthy male subjects. Aliment Pharmacol Ther. 2015;41(7):636–48. https://doi.org/10.1111/apt.13121.
51. Laine L, DeVault K, Katz P, et al. Vonoprazan versus lansoprazole for healing and maintenance of healing of erosive esophagitis: a randomized trial. Gastroenterology. 2023;164(1):61–71. https://doi.org/10.1053/j.gastro.2022.09.041.
52. Agago DE, Hanif N, Ajay Kumar AS, et al. Comparison of potassium-competitive acid blockers and proton pump inhibitors in patients with gastroesophageal reflux disease: a systematic review and meta-analysis of randomized controlled trials. Cureus. 2024;16(7):e65141. https://doi.org/10.7759/cureus.65141.
53. Olbe L, Carlsson E, Lindberg P. A proton-pump inhibitor expedition: the case histories of omeprazole and esomeprazole. Nat Rev Drug Discov. 2003;2(2):132–9. https://doi.org/10.1038/nrd1010.
54. Khan M, Santana J, Donnellan C, Preston C, Moayyedi P. Medical treatments in the short term management of reflux oesophagitis. Cochrane Database Syst Rev. 2007;2:CD003244. https://doi.org/10.1002/14651858.CD003244.pub2.
55. Eriksson S, Långström G, Rikner L, Carlsson R, Naesdal J. Omeprazole and H2-receptor antagonists in the acute treatment of duodenal ulcer, gastric ulcer and reflux oesophagitis: a meta-analysis. Eur J Gastroenterol Hepatol. 1995;7(5):467–75.

56. Chiba N, De Gara CJ, Wilkinson JM, Hunt RH. Speed of healing and symptom relief in grade II to IV gastroesophageal reflux disease: a meta-analysis. Gastroenterology. 1997;112(6):1798–810.
57. Sigterman KE, van Pinxteren B, Bonis PA, Lau J, Numans ME. Short-term treatment with proton pump inhibitors, H2-receptor antagonists and prokinetics for gastro-oesophageal reflux disease-like symptoms and endoscopy negative reflux disease. Cochrane Database Syst Rev. 2013;5:CD002095. https://doi.org/10.1002/14651858.CD002095.pub5.
58. Strand DS, Kim D, Peura DA. 25 years of proton pump inhibitors: a comprehensive review. Gut Liver. 2017;11(1):27–37. https://doi.org/10.5009/gnl15502.
59. Shin JM, Sachs G. Pharmacology of proton pump inhibitors. Curr Gastroenterol Rep. 2008;10(6):528–34. https://doi.org/10.1007/s11894-008-0098-4.
60. Shin JM, Kim N. Pharmacokinetics and pharmacodynamics of the proton pump inhibitors. J Neurogastroenterol Motil. 2013;19(1):25–35. https://doi.org/10.5056/jnm.2013.19.1.25.
61. Metz DC, Ferron GM, Paul J, et al. Proton pump activation in stimulated parietal cells is regulated by gastric acid secretory capacity: a human study. J Clin Pharmacol. 2002;42(5):512–9. https://doi.org/10.1177/00912700222011562.
62. Wolfe MM, Sachs G. Acid suppression: optimizing therapy for gastroduodenal ulcer healing, gastroesophageal reflux disease, and stress-related erosive syndrome. Gastroenterology. 2000;118(2):S9–S31. https://doi.org/10.1016/S0016-5085(00)70004-7.
63. Castell D, Bagin R, Goldlust B, Major J, Hepburn B. Comparison of the effects of immediate-release omeprazole powder for oral suspension and pantoprazole delayed-release tablets on nocturnal acid breakthrough in patients with symptomatic gastro-oesophageal reflux disease. Aliment Pharmacol Ther. 2005;21(12):1467–74. https://doi.org/10.1111/j.1365-2036.2005.02513.x.
64. Katz PO, Koch FK, Ballard ED, et al. Comparison of the effects of immediate-release omeprazole oral suspension, delayed-release lansoprazole capsules and delayed-release esomeprazole capsules on nocturnal gastric acidity after bedtime dosing in patients with night-time GERD symptoms. Aliment Pharmacol Ther. 2007;25(2):197–205. https://doi.org/10.1111/j.1365-2036.2006.03191.x.
65. Howden CW. Review article: immediate-release proton-pump inhibitor therapy--potential advantages. Aliment Pharmacol Ther 2005;22 Suppl 3:25–30. doi:https://doi.org/10.1111/j.1365-2036.2005.02709.x.
66. Walker D, Ng Kwet Shing R, Jones D, Gruss HJ, Regula J. Challenges of correlating pH change with relief of clinical symptoms in gastro esophageal reflux disease: a phase III, randomized study of Zegerid versus Losec. PLoS One. 2015;10(2):e0116308. https://doi.org/10.1371/journal.pone.0116308.
67. Hassan-Alin M, Andersson T, Bredberg E, Röhss K. Pharmacokinetics of esomeprazole after oral and intravenous administration of single and repeated doses to healthy subjects. Eur J Clin Pharmacol. 2000;56(9–10):665–70. https://doi.org/10.1007/s002280000206.
68. Gralnek IM, Dulai GS, Fennerty MB, Spiegel BM. Esomeprazole versus other proton pump inhibitors in erosive esophagitis: a meta-analysis of randomized clinical trials. Clin Gastroenterol Hepatol. 2006;4(12):1452–8. https://doi.org/10.1016/j.cgh.2006.09.013.
69. Röhss K, Hasselgren G, Hedenström H. Effect of esomeprazole 40 mg vs omeprazole 40 mg on 24-hour intragastric pH in patients with symptoms of gastroesophageal reflux disease. Dig Dis Sci. 2002;47(5):954–8. https://doi.org/10.1023/a:1015009300955.
70. Miner P Jr, Katz PO, Chen Y, Sostek M. Gastric acid control with esomeprazole, lansoprazole, omeprazole, pantoprazole, and rabeprazole: a five-way crossover study. Am J Gastroenterol. 2003;98(12):2616–20. https://doi.org/10.1111/j.1572-0241.2003.08783.x.
71. Johnson DA, Stacy T, Ryan M, et al. A comparison of esomeprazole and lansoprazole for control of intragastric pH in patients with symptoms of gastro-oesophageal reflux disease. Aliment Pharmacol Ther. 2005;22(2):129–34. https://doi.org/10.1111/j.1365-2036.2005.02534.x.
72. Katz PO, Castell DO, Chen Y, Andersson T, Sostek MB. Intragastric acid suppression and pharmacokinetics of twice-daily esomeprazole: a randomized, three-way crossover study.

Aliment Pharmacol Ther. 2004;20(4):399–406. https://doi.org/10.1111/j.1365-2036.2004.02079.x.
73. Kalaitzakis E, Björnsson E. A review of esomeprazole in the treatment of gastroesophageal reflux disease (GERD). Ther Clin Risk Manag. 2007;3(4):653–63.
74. Mathews S, Reid A, Tian C, Cai Q. An update on the use of pantoprazole as a treatment for gastroesophageal reflux disease. Clin Exp Gastroenterol. 2010;3:11–6.
75. Jungnickel PW. Pantoprazole: a new proton pump inhibitor. Clin Ther. 2000;22(11):1268–93. https://doi.org/10.1016/s0149-2918(00)83025-8.
76. Sachs G, Shin JM. The basis of differentiation of PPIs. Drugs Today (Barc). 2004;40 Suppl A:9–14.
77. Richter JE, Bochenek W. Oral pantoprazole for erosive esophagitis: a placebo-controlled, randomized clinical trial. Pantoprazole US GERD Study Group. Am J Gastroenterol. 2000;95(11):3071–80. https://doi.org/10.1111/j.1572-0241.2000.03254.x.
78. Mulder CJJ, Westerveld BD, Smit JM, et al. A double-blind, randomized comparison of omeprazole Multiple Unit Pellet System (MUPS) 20 mg, lansoprazole 30 mg and pantoprazole 40 mg in symptomatic reflux oesophagitis followed by 3 months of omeprazole MUPS maintenance treatment: a Dutch multicentre trial. Eur J Gastroen Hepat. 2002;14(6):649–56. https://doi.org/10.1097/00042737-200206000-00010.
79. Thomson A. Impact of PPIs on patient focused symptomatology in GERD. Ther Clin Risk Manag. 2008;4(6):1185–200.
80. Scholten T, Gatz G, Hole U. Once-daily pantoprazole 40 mg and esomeprazole 40 mg have equivalent overall efficacy in relieving GERD-related symptoms. Aliment Pharmacol Ther. 2003;18(6):587–94. https://doi.org/10.1046/j.1365-2036.2003.01745.x.
81. Baldi F, Malfertheiner P. Lansoprazole fast disintegrating tablet: a new formulation for an established proton pump inhibitor. Digestion. 2003;67(1–2):1–5. https://doi.org/10.1159/000070393.
82. Frazzoni M, De Micheli E, Grisendi A, Savarino V. Lansoprazole vs. omeprazole for gastro-oesophageal reflux disease: a pH-metric comparison. Aliment Pharmacol Ther. 2002;16(1):35–9. https://doi.org/10.1046/j.1365-2036.2002.01138.x.
83. Hershcovici T, Jha LK, Fass R. Dexlansoprazole MR: a review. Ann Med. 2011;43(5):366–74. https://doi.org/10.3109/07853890.2011.554429.
84. Skrzydło-Radomańska B, Radwan P. Dexlansoprazole – a new-generation proton pump inhibitor. Prz Gastroenterol. 2015;10(4):191–6. https://doi.org/10.5114/pg.2015.56109.
85. Wu MS, Tan SC, Xiong T. Indirect comparison of randomised controlled trials: comparative efficacy of dexlansoprazole vs. esomeprazole in the treatment of gastro-oesophageal reflux disease. Aliment Pharmacol Ther. 2013;38(2):190–201. https://doi.org/10.1111/apt.12349.
86. Morelli G, Chen H, Rossiter G, Rege B, Lu Y. An open-label, parallel, multiple-dose study comparing the pharmacokinetics and gastric acid suppression of rabeprazole extended-release with esomeprazole 40 mg and rabeprazole delayed-release 20 mg in healthy volunteers. Aliment Pharmacol Ther. 2011;33(7):845–54. https://doi.org/10.1111/j.1365-2036.2011.04580.x.
87. Laine L, Katz PO, Johnson DA, et al. Randomised clinical trial: a novel rabeprazole extended release 50 mg formulation vs. esomeprazole 40 mg in healing of moderate-to-severe erosive oesophagitis – the results of two double-blind studies. Aliment Pharmacol Ther. 2011;33(2):203–12. https://doi.org/10.1111/j.1365-2036.2010.04516.x.
88. Ogawa R, Echizen H. Drug-drug interaction profiles of proton pump inhibitors. Clin Pharmacokinet. 2010;49(8):509–33. https://doi.org/10.2165/11531320-000000000-00000.
89. Wedemeyer RS, Blume H. Pharmacokinetic drug interaction profiles of proton pump inhibitors: an update. Drug Saf. 2014;37(4):201–11. https://doi.org/10.1007/s40264-014-0144-0.
90. O'Donoghue ML, Braunwald E, Antman EM, et al. Pharmacodynamic effect and clinical efficacy of clopidogrel and prasugrel with or without a proton-pump inhibitor: an analysis of two randomised trials. Lancet (London, England). 2009;374(9694):989–97. https://doi.org/10.1016/S0140-6736(09)61525-7.

91. Bhatt DL, Cryer BL, Contant CF, et al. Clopidogrel with or without omeprazole in coronary artery disease. N Engl J Med. 2010;363(20):1909–17. https://doi.org/10.1056/NEJMoa1007964.
92. Laine L, Hennekens C. Proton pump inhibitor and clopidogrel interaction: fact or fiction? Am J Gastroenterol. 2010;105(1):34–41. https://doi.org/10.1038/ajg.2009.638.
93. Moayyedi P, Eikelboom JW, Bosch J, et al. Safety of proton pump inhibitors based on a large, multi-year, randomized trial of patients receiving rivaroxaban or aspirin. Gastroenterology. 2019;157(3):682–691.e2. https://doi.org/10.1053/j.gastro.2019.05.056.
94. Yibirin M, De Oliveira D, Valera R, Plitt AE, Lutgen S. Adverse effects associated with proton pump inhibitor use. Cureus. 2021;13(1):e12759. https://doi.org/10.7759/cureus.12759.
95. Laheij RJ, Sturkenboom MC, Hassing RJ, Dieleman J, Stricker BH, Jansen JB. Risk of community-acquired pneumonia and use of gastric acid-suppressive drugs. JAMA. 2004;292(16):1955–60. https://doi.org/10.1001/jama.292.16.1955.
96. Lambert AA, Lam JO, Paik JJ, Ugarte-Gil C, Drummond MB, Crowell TA. Risk of community-acquired pneumonia with outpatient proton-pump inhibitor therapy: a systematic review and meta-analysis. PLoS One. 2015;10(6):e0128004. https://doi.org/10.1371/journal.pone.0128004.
97. Herzig SJ, Howell MD, Ngo LH, Marcantonio ER. Acid-suppressive medication use and the risk for hospital-acquired pneumonia. JAMA. 2009;301(20):2120–8. https://doi.org/10.1001/jama.2009.722.
98. Sarkar M, Hennessy S, Yang YX. Proton-pump inhibitor use and the risk for community-acquired pneumonia. Ann Intern Med. 2008;149(6):391–8. https://doi.org/10.7326/0003-4819-149-6-200809160-00005.
99. Othman F, Crooks CJ, Card TR. Community acquired pneumonia incidence before and after proton pump inhibitor prescription: population based study. BMJ. 2016;355:i5813. https://doi.org/10.1136/bmj.i5813.
100. Filion KB, Chateau D, Targownik LE, et al. Proton pump inhibitors and the risk of hospitalisation for community-acquired pneumonia: replicated cohort studies with meta-analysis. Gut. 2014;63(4):552–8. https://doi.org/10.1136/gutjnl-2013-304738.
101. Vaezi MF, Yang YX, Howden CW. Complications of proton pump inhibitor therapy. Gastroenterology. 2017;153(1):35–48. https://doi.org/10.1053/j.gastro.2017.04.047.
102. Su T, Lai S, Lee A, He X, Chen S. Meta-analysis: proton pump inhibitors moderately increase the risk of small intestinal bacterial overgrowth. J Gastroenterol. 2018;53(1):27–36. https://doi.org/10.1007/s00535-017-1371-9.
103. Lo WK, Chan WW. Proton pump inhibitor use and the risk of small intestinal bacterial overgrowth: a meta-analysis. Clin Gastroenterol Hepatol. 2013;11(5):483–90. https://doi.org/10.1016/j.cgh.2012.12.011.
104. Imhann F, Bonder MJ, Vich Vila A, et al. Proton pump inhibitors affect the gut microbiome. Gut. 2016;65(5):740–8. https://doi.org/10.1136/gutjnl-2015-310376.
105. Seto CT, Jeraldo P, Orenstein R, Chia N, DiBaise JK. Prolonged use of a proton pump inhibitor reduces microbial diversity: implications for Clostridium difficile susceptibility. Microbiome. 2014;2:42. https://doi.org/10.1186/2049-2618-2-42.
106. Jaynes M, Kumar AB. The risks of long-term use of proton pump inhibitors: a critical review. Ther Adv Drug Saf. 2019;10:2042098618809927. https://doi.org/10.1177/2042098618809927.
107. Freedberg DE, Salmasian H, Friedman C, Abrams JA. Proton pump inhibitors and risk for recurrent Clostridium difficile infection among inpatients. Am J Gastroenterol. 2013;108(11):1794–801. https://doi.org/10.1038/ajg.2013.333.
108. Trifan A, Stanciu C, Girleanu I, et al. Proton pump inhibitors therapy and risk of Clostridium difficile infection: systematic review and meta-analysis. World J Gastroenterol. 2017;23(35):6500–15. https://doi.org/10.3748/wjg.v23.i35.6500.
109. Freedberg DE, Kim LS, Yang YX. The risks and benefits of long-term use of proton pump inhibitors: expert review and best practice advice from the American Gastroenterological

Association. Gastroenterology. 2017;152(4):706–15. https://doi.org/10.1053/j.gastro.2017.01.031.

110. Lam JR, Schneider JL, Zhao W, Corley DA. Proton pump inhibitor and histamine 2 receptor antagonist use and vitamin B12 deficiency. JAMA. 2013;310(22):2435–42. https://doi.org/10.1001/jama.2013.280490.
111. Lam JR, Schneider JL, Quesenberry CP, Corley DA. Proton pump inhibitor and histamine-2 receptor antagonist use and iron deficiency. Gastroenterology. 2017;152(4):821–829.e1. https://doi.org/10.1053/j.gastro.2016.11.023.
112. Tran-Duy A, Connell NJ, Vanmolkot FH, et al. Use of proton pump inhibitors and risk of iron deficiency: a population-based case-control study. J Intern Med. 2019;285(2):205–14. https://doi.org/10.1111/joim.12826.
113. Bezwoda W, Charlton R, Bothwell T, Torrance J, Mayet F. The importance of gastric hydrochloric acid in the absorption of nonheme food iron. J Lab Clin Med. 1978;92(1):108–16.
114. Liao S, Gan L, Mei Z. Does the use of proton pump inhibitors increase the risk of hypomagnesemia: an updated systematic review and meta-analysis. Medicine (Baltimore). 2019;98(13):e15011. https://doi.org/10.1097/MD.0000000000015011.
115. Hess MW, Hoenderop JG, Bindels RJ, Drenth JP. Systematic review: hypomagnesaemia induced by proton pump inhibition. Aliment Pharmacol Ther. 2012;36(5):405–13. https://doi.org/10.1111/j.1365-2036.2012.05201.x.
116. Yang YX. Chronic proton pump inihibitor therapy and calcium metabolism. Curr Gastroenterol Rep. 2012;14(6):473–9. https://doi.org/10.1007/s11894-012-0290-4.
117. Zhou B, Huang Y, Li H, Sun W, Liu J. Proton-pump inhibitors and risk of fractures: an update meta-analysis. Osteoporos Int. 2016;27(1):339–47. https://doi.org/10.1007/s00198-015-3365-x.
118. Ngamruengphong S, Leontiadis GI, Radhi S, Dentino A, Nugent K. Proton pump inhibitors and risk of fracture: a systematic review and meta-analysis of observational studies. Am J Gastroenterol. 2011;106(7):1209–18; quiz 1219. https://doi.org/10.1038/ajg.2011.113.
119. Nassar Y, Richter S. Proton-pump inhibitor use and fracture risk: an updated systematic review and meta-analysis. J Bone Metab. 2018;25(3):141–51. https://doi.org/10.11005/jbm.2018.25.3.141.
120. Corley DA, Kubo A, Zhao W, Quesenberry C. Proton pump inhibitors and histamine-2 receptor antagonists are associated with hip fractures among at-risk patients. Gastroenterology. 2010;139(1):93–101. https://doi.org/10.1053/j.gastro.2010.03.055.
121. Khalili H, Huang ES, Jacobson BC, Camargo CA, Feskanich D, Chan AT. Use of proton pump inhibitors and risk of hip fracture in relation to dietary and lifestyle factors: a prospective cohort study. BMJ. 2012;344:e372.
122. Aleraij S, Alhowti S, Ferwana M, Abdulmajeed I. Effect of proton pump inhibitors on bone mineral density: a systematic review and meta-analysis of observational studies. Bone Rep. 2020;13:100732. https://doi.org/10.1016/j.bonr.2020.100732.
123. Hussain S, Singh A, Zameer S, et al. No association between proton pump inhibitor use and risk of dementia: evidence from a meta-analysis. J Gastroenterol Hepatol. 2020;35(1):19–28. https://doi.org/10.1111/jgh.14789.
124. Xie Y, Bowe B, Li T, Xian H, Balasubramanian S, Al-Aly Z. Proton pump inhibitors and risk of incident CKD and progression to ESRD. J Am Soc Nephrol. 2016;27(10):3153–63. https://doi.org/10.1681/ASN.2015121377.
125. Blank ML, Parkin L, Paul C, Herbison P. A nationwide nested case-control study indicates an increased risk of acute interstitial nephritis with proton pump inhibitor use. Kidney Int. 2014;86(4):837–44. https://doi.org/10.1038/ki.2014.74.
126. Hart E, Dunn TE, Feuerstein S, Jacobs DM. Proton pump inhibitors and risk of acute and chronic kidney disease: a retrospective cohort study. Pharmacotherapy. 2019;39(4):443–53. https://doi.org/10.1002/phar.2235.
127. Klatte DCF, Gasparini A, Xu H, et al. Association between proton pump inhibitor use and risk of progression of chronic kidney disease. Gastroenterology. 2017;153(3):702–10. https://doi.org/10.1053/j.gastro.2017.05.046.

128. Lazarus B, Chen Y, Wilson FP, et al. Proton pump inhibitor use and the risk of chronic kidney disease. JAMA Intern Med. 2016;176(2):238–46. https://doi.org/10.1001/jamainternmed.2015.7193.
129. Xie Y, Bowe B, Li T, Xian H, Yan Y, Al-Aly Z. Long-term kidney outcomes among users of proton pump inhibitors without intervening acute kidney injury. Kidney Int. 2017;91(6):1482–94. https://doi.org/10.1016/j.kint.2016.12.021.
130. Sierra F, Suarez M, Rey M, Vela MF. Systematic review: proton pump inhibitor-associated acute interstitial nephritis. Aliment Pharmacol Ther. 2007;26(4):545–53. https://doi.org/10.1111/j.1365-2036.2007.03407.x.
131. Gomm W, von Holt K, Thomé F, et al. Association of Proton Pump Inhibitors with Risk of dementia: a Pharmacoepidemiological claims data analysis. JAMA Neurol. 2016;73(4):410–6. https://doi.org/10.1001/jamaneurol.2015.4791.
132. Badiola N, Alcalde V, Pujol A, et al. The proton-pump inhibitor lansoprazole enhances amyloid beta production. PLoS One. 2013;8(3):e58837. https://doi.org/10.1371/journal.pone.0058837.
133. Taipale H, Tolppanen AM, Tiihonen M, Tanskanen A, Tiihonen J, Hartikainen S. No association between proton pump inhibitor use and risk of Alzheimer's disease. Am J Gastroenterol. 2017;112(12):1802–8. https://doi.org/10.1038/ajg.2017.196.
134. Lochhead P, Hagan K, Joshi AD, et al. Association between proton pump inhibitor use and cognitive function in women. Gastroenterology. 2017;153(4):971–979.e4. https://doi.org/10.1053/j.gastro.2017.06.061.
135. Hsu PI, Lu CL, Wu DC, et al. Eight weeks of esomeprazole therapy reduces symptom relapse, compared with 4 weeks, in patients with Los Angeles grade A or B erosive esophagitis. Clin Gastroenterol Hepatol. 2015;13(5):859–66.e1. https://doi.org/10.1016/j.cgh.2014.09.033.
136. Spechler SJ, Hunter JG, Jones KM, et al. Randomized trial of Medical versus surgical treatment for refractory heartburn. N Engl J Med. 2019;381(16):1513–23. https://doi.org/10.1056/NEJMoa1811424.
137. Scarpellini E, Ang D, Pauwels A, De Santis A, Vanuytsel T, Tack J. Management of refractory typical GERD symptoms. Nat Rev Gastroenterol Hepatol. 2016;13(5):281–94. https://doi.org/10.1038/nrgastro.2016.50.
138. Graham DY, Tansel A. Interchangeable use of proton pump inhibitors based on relative potency. Clin Gastroenterol Hepatol. 2018;16(6):800–808.e7. https://doi.org/10.1016/j.cgh.2017.09.033.
139. Miehlke S, Lobe S, Madisch A, et al. Intragastric acidity during administration of generic omeprazole or esomeprazole – a randomised, two-way crossover study including CYP2C19 genotyping. Aliment Pharm Therap. 2011;33(4):471–6. https://doi.org/10.1111/j.1365-2036.2010.04544.x.
140. McRorie JW Jr, Gibb RD, Miner PB Jr. Evidence-based treatment of frequent heartburn: the benefits and limitations of over-the-counter medications. J Am Assoc Nurse Pract. 2014;26(6):330–9. https://doi.org/10.1002/2327-6924.12133.
141. Fass R, Sontag SJ, Traxler B, Sostek M. Treatment of patients with persistent heartburn symptoms: a double-blind, randomized trial. Clin Gastroenterol Hepatol. 2006;4(1):50–6.
142. Mainie I, Tutuian R, Shay S, et al. Acid and non-acid reflux in patients with persistent symptoms despite acid suppressive therapy: a multicentre study using combined ambulatory impedance-pH monitoring. Gut. 2006;55(10):1398–402. https://doi.org/10.1136/gut.2005.087668.
143. Fass R, Murthy U, Hayden CW, et al. Omeprazole 40 mg once a day is equally effective as lansoprazole 30 mg twice a day in symptom control of patients with gastro-oesophageal reflux disease (GERD) who are resistant to conventional-dose lansoprazole therapy-a prospective, randomized, multi-centre study. Aliment Pharmacol Ther. 2000;14(12):1595–603.
144. Farrell B, Pottie K, Thompson W, et al. Deprescribing proton pump inhibitors: evidence-based clinical practice guideline. Can Fam Physician. 2017;63(5):354–64.
145. Inadomi JM, Jamal R, Murata GH, et al. Step-down management of gastroesophageal reflux disease. Gastroenterology. 2001;121(5):1095–100.

146. Bate CM, Booth SN, Crowe JP, et al. Omeprazole 10 mg or 20 mg once daily in the prevention of recurrence of reflux oesophagitis. Solo Investigator Group. Gut. 1995;36(4):492–8. https://doi.org/10.1136/gut.36.4.492.
147. Tsuzuki T, Okada H, Kawahara Y, et al. Proton pump inhibitor step-down therapy for GERD: a multi-center study in Japan. World J Gastroenterol. 2011;17(11):1480–7. https://doi.org/10.3748/wjg.v17.i11.1480.

Laparoscopic Anti-reflux Surgery

Francisco Schlottmann, José Barros Sosa, Rudolf Buxhoeveden, Fernando A. M. Herbella, and Marco G. Patti

Introduction

Gastroesophageal reflux disease (GERD) represents one of the most frequent gastrointestinal disorders. It is estimated that approximately 20% of adults in Western populations are affected. Although the majority of patients achieve adequate symptom control through lifestyle changes and pharmacological therapy, a subset will ultimately require surgical intervention. Surgery should be considered in patients who present with persistent symptoms despite medication (such as recurrent regurgitation), large hiatal hernias, poor adherence to medical treatment, reluctance to maintain long-term pharmacotherapy, or adverse effects from medications.

Relying solely on clinical symptoms for the diagnosis of GERD can often lead to misdiagnosis, given its variable presentation and overlap with other gastrointestinal disorders. Therefore, prior to any surgical intervention, we recommend confirming the diagnosis through upper endoscopy, barium swallow study, high-resolution manometry, and pH monitoring.

Successful anti-reflux surgery relies heavily on appropriate patient selection, comprehensive preoperative assessment, and meticulous surgical technique [1–5].

F. Schlottmann (✉)
University of Buenos Aires, Ciudad Autónoma Buenos Aires, Buenos Aires, Argentina

J. B. Sosa · R. Buxhoeveden
Department of Surgery, Hospital Alemán of Buenos Aires, Buenos Aires, Argentina
e-mail: jbarros@hospitalaleman.com; rbuxhoeveden@hospitalaleman.com

F. A. M. Herbella
Department of Surgery, Federal University of São Paulo, São Paulo, São Paulo, Brazil
e-mail: herbella.dcir@epm.br

M. G. Patti
Department of Surgery, University of Virginia Hospital, Charlottesville, VA, USA

F. Schlottmann et al. (eds.), *Esophageal Disorders*,
https://doi.org/10.1007/978-3-032-08179-7_4

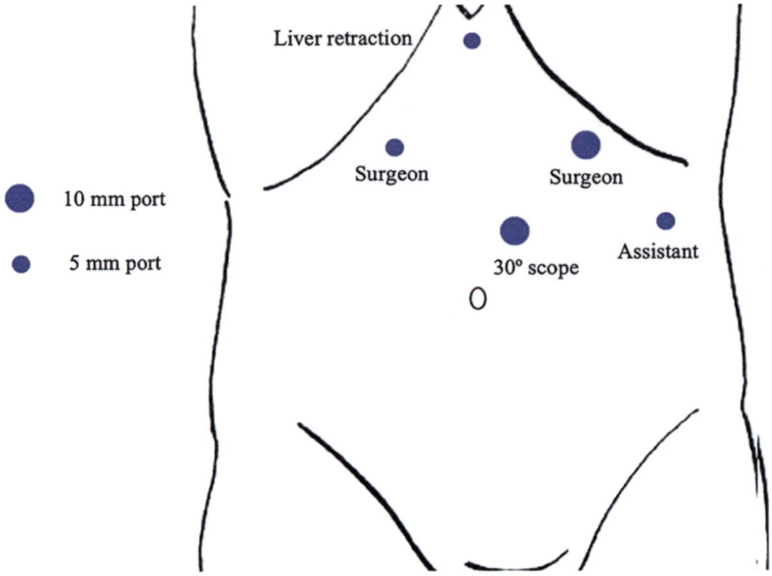

Fig. 1 Ports placement for laparoscopic antireflux surgery

Surgical Technique

Patient Positioning and Trocar Placement

The patient is positioned in a low lithotomy setup, with legs extended in stirrups and knees flexed approximately 20°–30°. Pneumatic compression devices are strongly advised to minimize the risk of deep vein thrombosis. Throughout the procedure, the surgeon operates standing between the patient's legs. Typically, five laparoscopic ports are utilized (two 10-mm and three 5-mm) (Fig. 1).

Division of the Short Gastric Vessels

Using a vessel-sealing device, the short gastric vessels are divided, beginning midway along the greater curvature of the stomach and extending toward the gastric fundus (Fig. 2). Dissection continues up to the left crus (Fig. 3). This step will facilitate obtaining a tension-free fundoplication later in the procedure. For patients with hiatal hernia (most patients undergoing anti-reflux), resection of the hernia sac is recommended (Fig. 4).

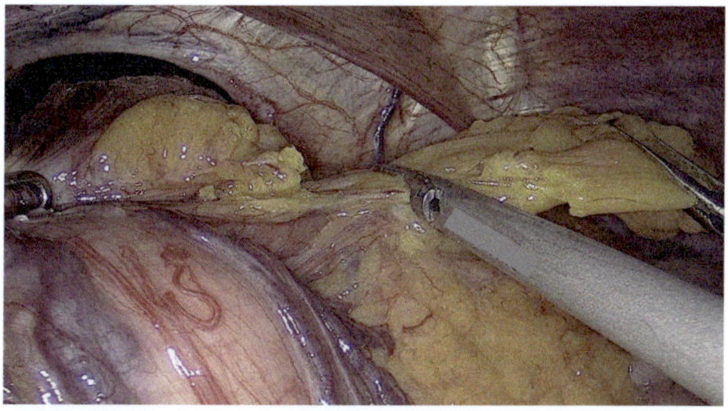

Fig. 2 Division of short gastric vessels

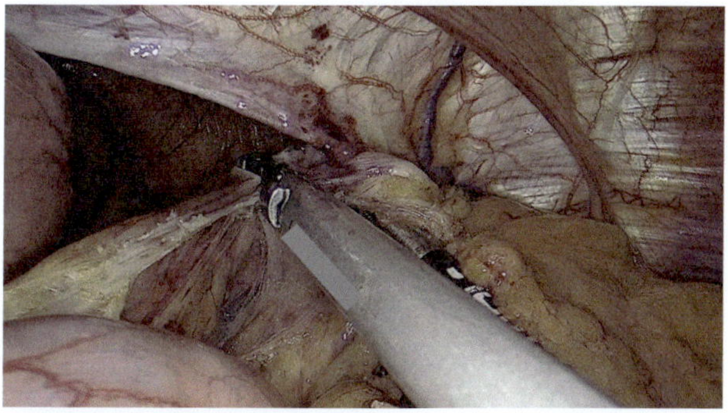

Fig. 3 Dissection of the left crus

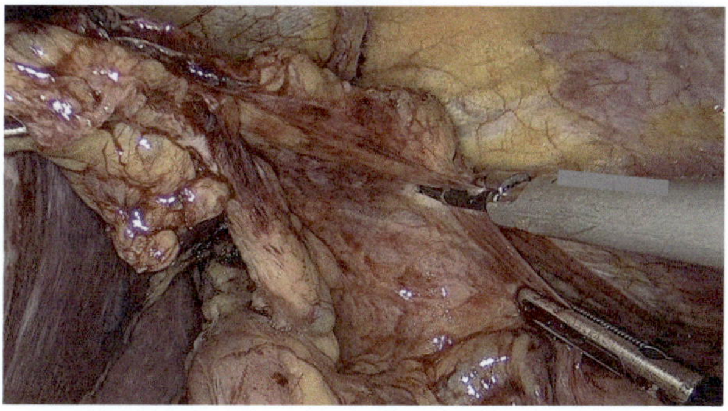

Fig. 4 Resection of hernia sac

Division of the Phrenoesophageal Membrane

After full dissection of the left crus, the phrenoesophageal membrane is incised just above the esophagus. The anterior vagus nerve must be carefully identified and preserved by keeping it attached to the esophageal wall. Gentle blunt dissection is performed to separate the esophagus from its anterior mediastinal and left crus attachments.

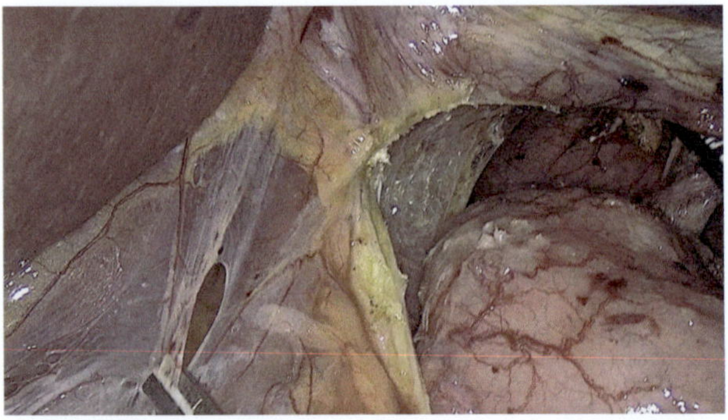

Fig. 5 Division of the gastrohepatic ligament

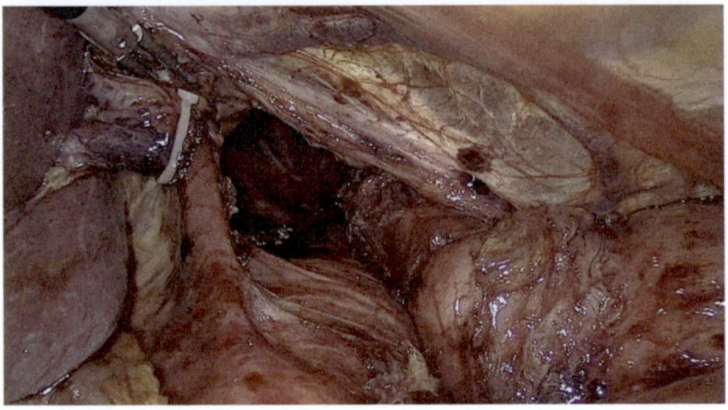

Fig. 6 Dissection of the right crus

Division of the Gastrohepatic Ligament

The gastrohepatic ligament is dissected using electrocautery or an ultrasonic device, starting above the caudate lobe of the liver and progressing toward the right crus (Fig. 5). The right crus is subsequently dissected down to its junction with the left crus (Fig. 6), allowing further mobilization of the esophagus by gentle blunt maneuvers. The posterior vagus nerve must be visualized and preserved during this step.

Mediastinal Dissection

Following complete mobilization from the crura, a posterior window beneath the esophagus is created with blunt dissection (Fig. 7). This space is widened to permit passage of a Penrose drain or umbilical tape around the esophagus, which is secured and used to retract the esophagus away from the hiatus. This maneuver greatly facilitates an extensive mediastinal dissection, ensuring at least 3 cm of intra-abdominal esophagus is obtained (Fig. 8).

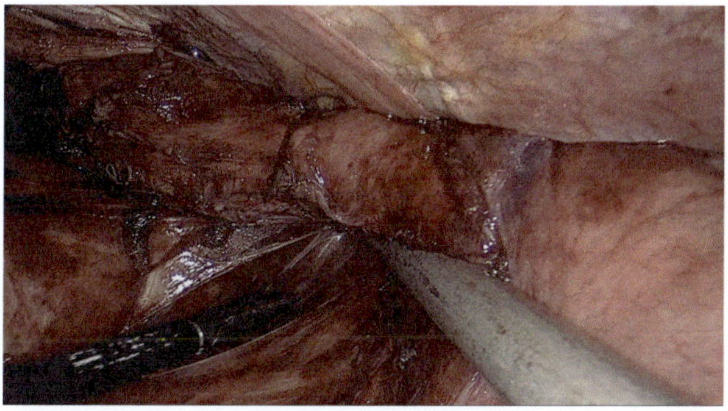

Fig. 7 Posterior window under the esophagus

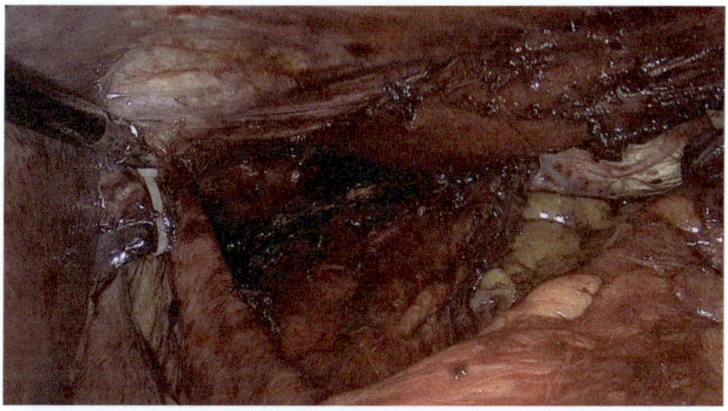

Fig. 8 Complete mediastinal dissection with at least 3 cm of esophagus under the diaphragm

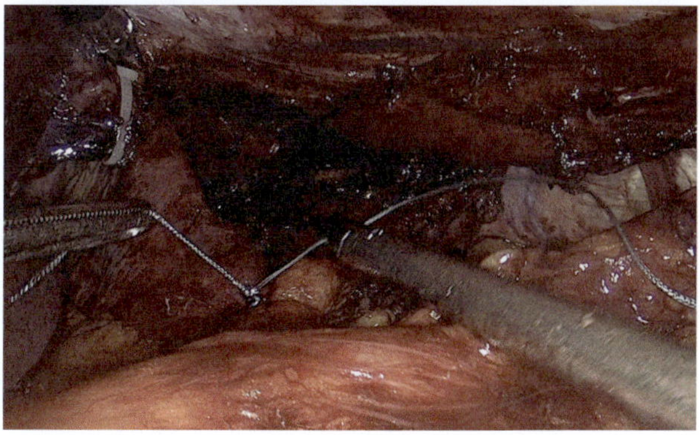

Fig. 9 Closure of the hiatus with interrupted non-absorbable sutures

Closure of the Esophageal Hiatus

The esophageal hiatus is clearly exposed by upward and leftward retraction of the esophagus. The right and left crus are approximated with interrupted non-absorbable sutures (e.g., 2-0 silk or polyester), starting just above the junction of the pillars and proceeding superiorly at 1-cm intervals. Closure should avoid excessive tightness to prevent postoperative dysphagia; a closed grasper should pass comfortably between the esophagus and the sutures (Figs. 9 and 10).

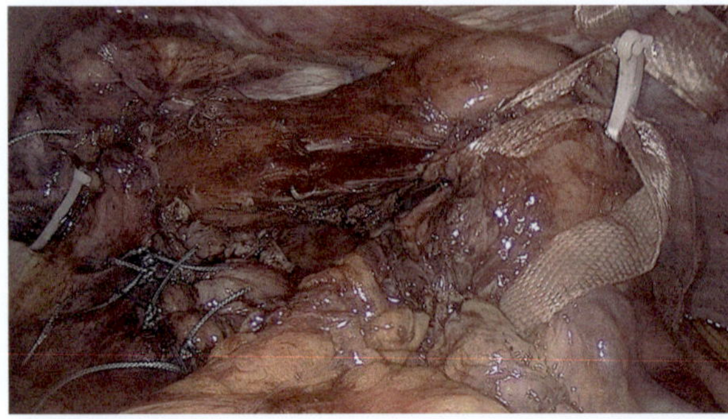

Fig. 10 The hiatus is satisfactorily closed

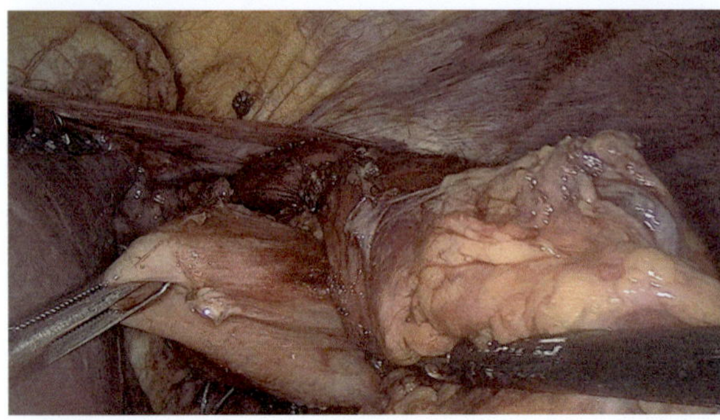

Fig. 11 The gastric fundus is passed posteriorly around the esophagus

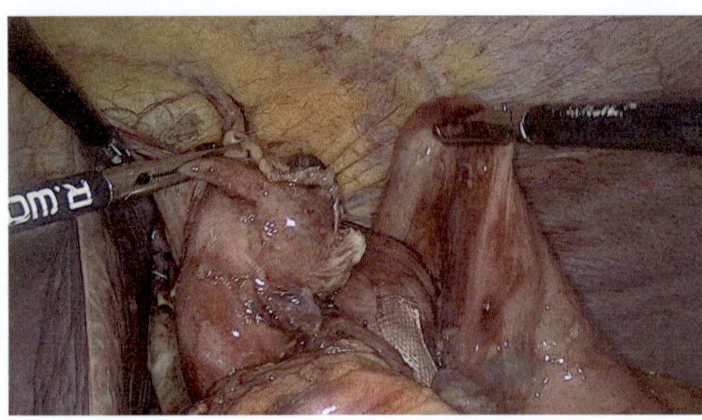

Fig. 12 "Shoe shine" maneuver

Fundoplication

After adequate crural closure, the gastric fundus is passed posteriorly around the esophagus and a "shoe-shine" maneuver is performed to verify sufficient mobilization (Figs. 11 and 12). A complete 360° fundoplication (Nissen) is generally performed. A bougie or the endoscope is preferably introduced into the esophagus before constructing the wrap to help prevent postoperative dysphagia. Graspers are used to hold the fundus on either side of the gastroesophageal junction during placement of the first stitch. Usually, three sutures spaced 1 cm apart are used to create a short (approximately 2 cm) and floppy wrap (Fig. 13).

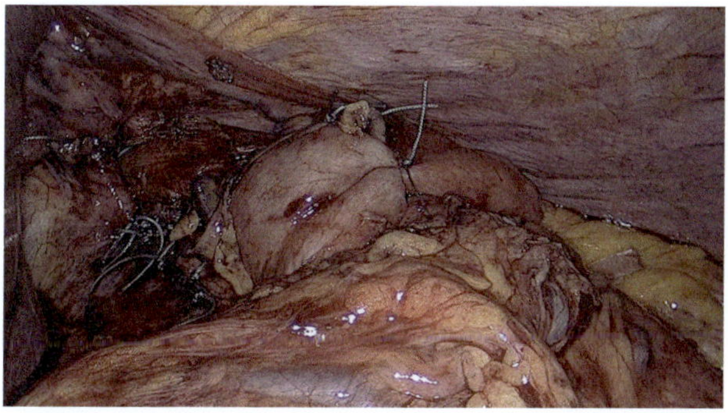

Fig. 13 Completed Nissen fundoplication

In cases of significant esophageal motility disorders, a partial fundoplication is recommended.

Final Inspection

The bougie is removed by the anesthesiologist, and the Penrose drain is cut and extracted. We often perform intraoperative endoscopy to confirm that the gastro-esophageal junction is not excessively tight and to inspect the fundoplication from the inside. All trocars are removed under direct vision with careful hemostasis control, and fascial closure is performed for all 10–12 mm port sites.

Postoperative Care

Patients can initiate a clear liquid diet on the day of surgery and advance to a soft diet as tolerated. Most individuals are discharged within 48 hours postoperatively. Anti-reflux medications are typically discontinued around 4 weeks after surgery.

Conflict of Interest The authors have no conflicts of interest.

References

1. El-Serag HN, Sweet S, Winchester CC, et al. Update on the epidemiology of gastro-esophageal reflux disease: a systematic review. Gut. 2014;63:871–80.
2. Schlottmann F, Herbella FA, Allaix ME, et al. Surgical treatment of gastroesophageal reflux disease. World J Surg. 2017;41(7):1685–90.
3. Schlottmann F, Strassle PD, Patti MG. Antireflux surgery in the USA: influence of surgical volume on perioperative outcomes and costs – time for centralization? World J Surg. 2018;42(7):2183–9.
4. Patti MG, Schlottmann F, Farrell TM. Fundoplication for gastroesophageal reflux disease: tips for success. J Laparoendosc Adv Surg Tech A. 2017;27(1):1–5.
5. Patti MG, Schlottmann F. Recurrence of reflux after laparoscopic antireflux surgery. JAMA. 2018;319(1):82–3.

Endoscopic Therapies for Gastroesophageal Reflux Disease

Sullivan A. Ayuso and Michael B. Ujiki

Introduction

Gastroesophageal reflux disease (GERD) is one of the most common medical conditions affecting quality of life. Approximately 20–30% of people worldwide are living with GERD, and this incidence is increasing with time [1]. Risk factors for GERD include obesity, smoking, caffeine, and female gender [2]. The gastroesophageal (GE) reflux barrier is multifaceted and is comprised of the lower esophageal sphincter (LES), the crural diaphragm, and angle of His, and the phrenoesophageal ligament [3]. When there are alterations in any part of this barrier, then patients may be prone to developing GERD. For example, the presence of a hiatal hernia may lessen the efficacy of the LES since it requires intraabdominal pressure to properly function.

Traditionally, medical therapy with proton pump inhibitors (PPIs) and anti-reflux surgery (ARS) have been the mainstay treatments for GERD. In fact, the surgical management of GERD using fundoplication remains the gold standard for long-term GERD treatment. Patients undergoing partial or complete laparoscopic fundoplication, which have equivalent outcomes, remain satisfied with their operation and are reflux free in 80–95% of cases [4–6]. However, in select patients, novel endoscopic therapies for GERD have become viable treatment options. The endoscopic treatment of GERD may offer a number of advantages including faster recovery,

S. A. Ayuso (✉)
Division of Gastrointestinal and General Surgery, Department of Surgery, Endeavor Health, Evanston, IL, USA

Evanston Hospital, Grainger Center for Simulation and Innovation, Evanston, IL, USA

M. B. Ujiki
Division of Gastrointestinal and General Surgery, Department of Surgery, Endeavor Health, Evanston, IL, USA
e-mail: MUjiki@northshore.org

F. Schlottmann et al. (eds.), *Esophageal Disorders*,
https://doi.org/10.1007/978-3-032-08179-7_5

decreased length of hospital stay, and in most cases, it does not burn a bridge for ARS if endoscopic treatment fails [7]. This chapter will review the workup, diagnosis, and available endoscopic therapies for patients with GERD.

Clinical Symptoms

Patients with GERD may have symptoms that are categorized as "typical" or "atypical" [8]. Typical symptoms include heartburn and regurgitation; however, only about half of patients will report atypical symptoms. Atypical symptoms may be varied and include presentation with laryngitis, cough, post-nasal drip, or dental erosion. In the case of excess mucous production or post-nasal drip, patients frequently are referred to an otolaryngologist for evaluation first and have had a negative laryngoscopy. It is also prudent to ask about symptoms like nausea, bloating, and early satiety that may be consistent with concomitant gastroparesis. If gastroparesis is confirmed on a gastric emptying study, then a pyloric intervention (e.g., gastric per oral endoscopic myotomy or laparoscopic pyloroplasty) could first be performed to see if this helps reflux symptoms.

Endoscopic Findings Consistent with GERD

Upper endoscopy is one of the main tools used for diagnosing GERD. Historically, there have been four main diagnostic tests used for working up patients prior to performing an antireflux procedure: esophagogastroduodenoscopy (EGD), pH testing, esophagram, and manometry. There are hallmark findings seen on EGD that are consistent with GERD. The Los Angeles (LA) Classification of Esophagitis evaluates the degree of mucosal disruption of the esophagus in patients with erosive esophagitis [9]. The LA Classification grades the degree of mucosal disruption on an A to D scale, with A being the least severe and D being most severe (Table 1). The LA Classification system has been extensively validated and correlates closely with esophageal acid exposure.

Performing an EGD can provide other information in addition to mucosal disruption. For instance, it allows us to determine the relative looseness of the GE flap valve (i.e., Hill grade) or presence of a hiatal or paraesophageal hernia, which can

Table 1 Los Angeles Classification System

Los Angeles Grade	Description
Grade A	≥1 mucosal break, ≤5 mm, no extension between mucosal folds
Grade B	≥1 mucosal break, ≥5 mm, no extension between mucosal folds
Grade C	≥1 mucosal break, ≥5 mm, extends between mucosal folds but involves less than 75% of circumference
Grade D	≥1 mucosal break, ≥5 mm, extends between mucosal folds and involves more than 75% of circumference

be indicative of GERD [10]. Perhaps most importantly, it can help with diagnosis of any malignant or a pre-malignant lesion, especially in the setting of dysphagia. Barrett's esophagus (BE) is defined histologically by the presence of squamocolumnar metaplasia at the GE junction (GEJ). Patients with BE have an increased risk of developing esophageal adenocarcinoma with a yearly incidence between 0.2% and 0.5% [11]. BE can be identified by the presence of salmon-colored tongues of mucosa extending proximally into the esophagus. BE is reported using the Prague criteria, which takes into account the circumferential (C) and maximal (M) extent of involvement of BE, which are measured in centimeters (cm).

The American Society of Gastrointestinal Endoscopy (ASGE) recommends the use of advanced imaging techniques to properly diagnose BE [12]. Narrow-band imaging (NBI) is frequently used as an adjunct; NBI works by utilizing blue and green light wavelengths to detect early vascular and mucosal irregularities and enhances sensitivity of detecting BE and non-erosive disease [13]. Non-dysplastic BE is treated with antacid medication and endoscopic surveillance is performed every 3–5 years [14]. By contrast patients with dysplastic BE may be treated with endoscopic ablation and/or resection techniques. It may be necessary to perform multiple treatments prior to a return to endoscopic surveillance.

Chronic GERD can also lead to esophageal scarring and stricture. In cases where a stricture is seen on upper endoscopy, biopsy should be performed to rule out malignancy or eosinophilic esophagitis. PPIs can help to promote short-term healing in the setting of peptic stricture and lead to symptomatic relief in patients who are complaining of dysphagia [15].

Wireless pH Testing

EGD can also be used to place the probe (i.e., Bravo probe) used for wireless pH testing under direct supervision. The Bravo probe is placed 6 cm proximal to the GE junction. Wireless pH testing should be performed off of antacid therapy in the setting of unproven GERD [16]. It is our practice to hold PPIs 2 weeks prior to Bravo testing for all patients regardless of their symptoms. H2 blockers are held 3 days prior to testing. Patients may resume their PPI after the 96-h test, though 48-h tests may also be performed. How patients clinically respond to being off of their antacid medication can provide further diagnostic information to the physician.

The main parameter that is being measured by wireless pH testing is acid exposure time (AET). AET quantifies the amount of time that pH is below 4 and is a central part of modern diagnostic criteria. Other information gleaned from pH testing includes number of reflux episodes along with Symptom Association Probability (SAP) and Symptom Index (SI) [17]. The SAP measures whether symptoms and reflux occurred within 2 min of each other and then uses a 2 × 2 table to calculate the number of 2-min segments with and without symptoms and reflux. An SAP of >95% is considered positive. The SI is the percentage of symptom events that are related to reflux episodes; an SI of >50% is considered positive. The patient must have a positive SAP for an SI to be meaningful.

Diagnosis of GERD

The DeMeester score has conventionally been used to diagnose patients with GERD and guide treatment [18]. The DeMeester score was developed in the early 1970s and is a composite score that allows for a quantitative means of expressing acid exposure in the distal esophagus. Specifically, it is based on six factors: the total number of reflux episodes, the length of the longest reflux episode, the number of episodes greater than 5 min, total percentage of monitoring time with a pH <4, and the percentage of time with pH <4 in the upright and supine positions. This score serves as a useful adjunct for cases in which the endoscopic diagnosis of GERD is unclear. In addition, it has been used as a marker for severity of GERD that can be helpful for counselling patients.

The updated Lyons Consensus (2.0), which was developed by a working group of 20 physicians, has provided a modern definition of actionable GERD [19]. The Lyons Consensus makes the distinction between borderline and conclusive evidence for GERD based on endoscopic findings and the results of wireless pH or pH impedance studies (Table 2). Borderline criteria for GERD include LA Grade A esophagitis and an AET of 4–6% on 24-h studies or two or more days on a wireless pH study. If the total number of reflux episodes are between 40 and 80, then this would also meet criteria for a borderline test. By contrast, conclusive criteria for GERD are Grade B-D esophagitis, biopsy proven BE, a peptic esophageal stricture, or an AET ≥6% on 24-h studies or for more than 2 days on wireless pH studies. There are other adjunctive findings that may support a GERD diagnosis and include factors such as the presence of a hiatal hernia, hypotensive lower esophageal sphincter on manometry, and a total number of reflux episodes >80.

Amundson et al. compared outcomes for patients undergoing antireflux surgery (ARS) who met historical criteria for GERD (LA Grade C/D esophagitis, BE or a DeMeester score of ≥14.72) versus those who met new American Gastrointestinal Association (AGA) criteria for GERD [20, 21]. The AGA criteria were similar to the modified Lyons criteria and included patients with Grade B esophagitis and an AET of ≥6% on two or more days on a wireless pH test. The authors found that 24%

Table 2 Lyons 2.0 Consensus Criteria for GERD

Diagnosis of GERD	Characteristics
Borderline	Endoscopic Findings: Grade A Esophagitis Acid Exposure Time: 24-h: 4–6% Wireless: 2 or more days, 4–6%
Definitive	Endoscopic Findings: Grade B or above Esophagitis Changes consistent with Barrett's Esophagus Peptic Stricture Acid Exposure Time: 24-h: ≥6% Wireless: 2 or more days ≥6%

of patients met historic criteria only, indicating that the new guidelines excluded a portion of patients who would've previously been diagnosed and surgically treated for GERD. The cohort that met historical criteria only had more atypical GERD symptoms and worse reflux symptom index (RSI) scores at 2 years postop, indicating that AET may better be able to define who should undergo ARS.

Preprocedural Considerations

As is standard for all patients who are offered procedural therapy for GERD, we make sure that conclusive diagnostic reflux criteria are met prior to proceeding. If conclusive diagnostic criteria for GERD are not sufficiently met, then patients may actually have worse outcomes, especially in the setting of esophageal hypersensitivity [22]. In the setting of borderline GERD, maximum medical management is attempted, and in some cases neuromodulation, prior to embarking on endoscopic treatment. An extensive risk and benefit conversation is had with patients and alternative medical and surgical treatment options are presented. Review of procedural outcomes, including institutional data, are discussed with patients so that they have an idea of what to expect following endoscopic intervention.

Transoral Incisionless Fundoplication (TIF) and Concomitant TIF (cTIF)

Technique and Key Steps

The TIF (now TIF 2.0) procedure allows endoscopists to create a 3–4 cm rotational wrap, mimicking a fundoplication, utilizing the cardia and the fundus of the stomach. It is most often perform using the EsophyXZ+ (EndoGastric Solutions, Inc., Redmond, WA, US). Patients are candidates for the procedure if they have a hiatal hernia that is less than or equal to 2 cm and a Hill grade valve of two or less [23]. Other contraindications to the procedure include esophageal obstruction or strictures, esophageal varices, limited neck mobility and LA Grade C and D esophagitis [24]. Unlike the aforementioned procedure, TIF must be performed under general anesthesia and not conscious sedation.

The EsophyXZ+ has an 18 mm frame, which allows a standard gastroscope to be placed through the device. A full endoscopy is conducted prior to the procedure to ensure the patient does not have any contraindications to TIF. The scope and the TIF device are introduced simultaneously and the scope is retroflexed to identify the GEJ and confirm proper location of the device. The helical retractor is used to grab tissue distal to the squamocolumnar junction and then the entire device is pulled back to ensure that the stomach engaged in the helix wraps around the esophagus in the direction of the lesser curvature. Once it is confirmed that the device is in the correct location and below the diaphragm, the polypropylene fasteners are fired between the stomach and the esophagus. The process is repeated in order to create a plication that is between 270° and 320°. Patients are discharged on an advancing esophageal diet and off of antacid medication.

The cTIF procedure has gained recent popularity and combines the TIF procedure with surgical closure of the hiatus. This allows surgeons to perform a TIF when there is a hiatal hernia that is greater than 2 cm. This procedure may be performed by a surgeon or in conjunction with a gastroenterologist who is present in the operating room. Proponents of the c-TIF procedure cite reproducibility of the fundoplication along with less gas bloat and dysphagia compared to traditional fundoplication [25].

Potential Pitfalls

Ensuring proper patient selection is critical to achieving the desired outcomes for TIF. If the TIF apparatus is applied to patients with a large hiatal hernia, this can be dangerous for patients as the plication may inadvertently be performed above the level of the diaphragm and damage intrathoracic structures. If any resistance is felt when passing the TIF device into the esophagus, then it should not be forced further. A jaw thrust may be needed and the device must be thoroughly lubricated. Occasionally, some endoscopists perform dilation prior to device placement in order to ensure that it passes easily. Fasteners should not be placed over each other during the procedure as this can also increase the risk of perforation. If there is any evidence of persistent bleeding from mucosal disruption, this should be addressed prior to terminating the TIF.

Outcomes

TIF was first introduced in 2000 and has amassed more data than other endoscopic treatment options for GERD. However, much of the data that is available for TIF includes different generations of TIF devices making it hard to interpret the existing literature. There are currently three published randomized controlled trials (RCTs) evaluating the efficacy of TIF 2.0. Each of these trials compared TIF to PPI or sham treatment. A meta-analysis of these RCTs showed that TIF significantly reduced PPI utilization, decreased acid exposure in the distal esophagus, and improved patient quality of life. In each of these trials, 59–90% of patients were off of PPIs at 6 months. Trad et al. subsequently published the 5-year results of one of these RCTs, the TEMPO Trial, which showed that 86% of patients remained regurgitation free while 66% remained off of PPIs [26]. The results of this study suggest durability of the TIF procedure.

There are no RCTs comparing outcomes of ARS to TIF or cTIF. Only one systematic review has attempted to evaluate outcomes of RCTs comparing fundoplication (specifically Nissen) and TIF to PPI and sham [27]. This review included seven total studies and demonstrated that fundoplication had a higher probability of increasing LES pressure and eliminating esophagitis but TIF had a higher probability of improving HRQL. Regression analysis indicated that a confounder contributing to this difference in HRQL was degree of follow-up. Patients who underwent TIF had shorter mean follow-up compared to those undergoing fundoplication.

Outcomes for cTIF are limited to observational studies. Jaber et al. recently published a systematic review of cTIF, which included seven retrospective studies [25]. In this study, nearly three quarters of patients reported being off of PPIs at up to 20 months follow-up. The rate of dysphagia and gas bloat were 5.3% and 6.9%, respectively. It is also difficult to study cTIF as there is marked variability in how people perform hiatal closure. With the advent of impedance planimetry, surgeons are able to tailor the tightness of crural closure and fundoplication, which may lead to less gas bloat and dysphagia regardless of the type of fundoplication that is performed [28].

Anti-reflux Mucosectomy (ARMS)

Technique and Key Steps

The ARMS procedure utilizes hemi-circumferential endoscopic mucosal resection (EMR) or endoscopic submucosal dissection (ESD) of the gastric cardia, near the GEJ, to induce scarring at the flap valve [29]. The tightening of the valve helps to prevent reflux of acid into the distal esophagus. The main contraindication to this procedure is the presence of a hiatal hernia greater than 2 cm. Prior to the procedure, manometry is performed to rule out an underlying major motility disorder.

The authors prefer to perform the procedure using a band-EMR technique. A Captivator EMR (Boston Scientific, Marlborough, MA) device is fastened to end of a standard GIF HQ190 upper endoscope (Olympus, Tokyo, Japan). The procedure is completed in a retroflexed manner and is started along the greater curvature of the stomach. A saline lift is performed prior to banding of the mucosa. Once a submucosal lift has been achieved, suction is used to draw the mucosa of the cardia into the EMR cap. Suction is applied for 10–15 s, and the desired "red-out" is seen, before firing the band. After the band has been fired, the tissue is resected just underneath the band using hot snare polypectomy.

These steps are repeatedly sequentially sparing two caps along the greater curvature and one cap along the lesser curvature (Fig. 1). The specimens are removed using a Roth net and then sent to pathology. The banded areas should be contiguous and if there are any mucosal areas that have not been resected, then argon plasma coagulation (APC) can be applied to the connecting mucosa. Patients are sent home the day of the procedure and PPIs are held. Carafate is not used in the postoperative setting as the intention is to promote scarring rather than mucosal healing. There is no significant dietary modification required post-procedure.

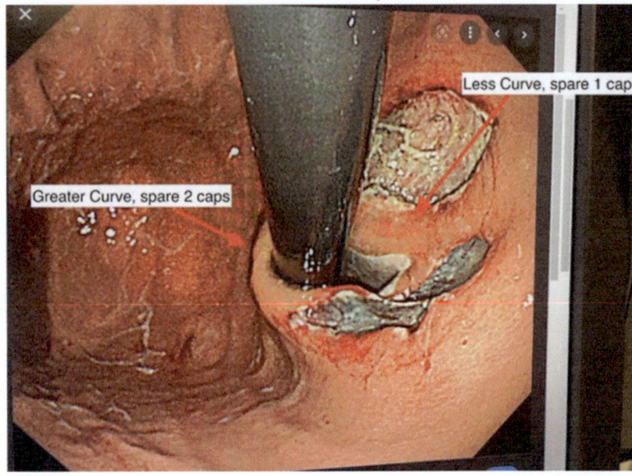

Fig. 1 Anti-reflux Mucosectomy (ARMS). The ARMS procedure utilizes band endoscopic mucosal resection or endoscopic submucosal dissection to target the gastric cardia around the gastroesophageal junction. It is our practice to spare two band EMR caps along the greater curvature and one cap along the lesser curvature

Potential Pitfalls

If EMR is carried onto the esophageal mucosa, then this can lead to stricture at the GEJ and resulting dysphagia. In this setting, patients may benefit from balloon dilation to alleviate symptoms. More acutely, when performing EMR, it is important to obtain a definitive submucosal lift prior to performing the resection. If an adequate lift is not achieved, then patients are at risk for perforation. When a perforation is suspected, it is critical to look closely at the area where EMR was performed. This may involve aggressively suctioning or irrigating the area to get an appropriate view. If perforation is confirmed, then there are a number of endoscopic options for repair, including the use of clips or endoscopic suturing. Only 0.4–0.7% of perforations happen in a delayed fashion, so it is important to have a high index of suspicion at the time of the procedure [21].

Outcomes

The ARMS technique was first introduced in 2014 by Inoue's group after incidentally noting improvement in reflux symptoms for a patient who underwent EMR for BE [30]. The group described the technique using either cap-assisted EMR or ESD. They demonstrated a mean improvement in DeMeester score by 5.2 and decreased mean AET from 29.1% to 3.1%. Since then, there have been a number of studies demonstrating similarly favorable results. Our group reported our early results for 19 patients using band EMR and found that nearly 70% of patients had improvement in GERD symptoms and were off of PPIs [29]. However, three of these patients did develop stricture and required ballon dilation, which may have been related to performing EMR to close to the GEJ.

Larger studies, such as the one by Sumi et al. (n = 109 patients), have reported that about half of patients undergoing ARMS are able to discontinue PPIs [31]. In that study, there were significant decreases in both DeMeester score and AET, but there was no difference in the number of proximal reflux events. A recent systematic review and meta-analysis reported a technical and clinical success rate of 97.7% and 80.1%, respectively [32]. There were significant improvements seen on GERD-HRQL (mean difference = 14.9) and GERD symptom questionnaire (mean difference = 4.9). The rate of post-procedure dysphagia remains approximately 10%. There are no prospective RCTs comparing ARMS to ARS; however retrospective reviews have found shorter length of stay, decreased postoperative pain, and faster return to activity with minimal or no difference in reflux symptom control [33, 34].

Anti-reflux Mucosal Ablation (ARMA)

Technique and Key Steps

The ARMA procedure has emerged as a viable alternative to the ARMS procedure. The intent of the procedure is the same as ARMS, which is to promote scarring around the GE flap valve and prevent backflow of acid into the distal esophagus. Once again, a hiatal hernia >2 cm is a contraindication and manometry is performed prior to the procedure. Instead of EMR or ESD, ablation is performed with APC in the same hemi-circumferential distribution (Fig. 2). The width of the ablation is approximately 1.5 cm. Typical APC settings are a flow of 0.8 L/min at a power range of 50–80 W. Our group has begun using this procedure in patient populations where surgical management of reflux may be difficult to achieve, such as in patients who continue to have reflux following a gastric bypass procedure.

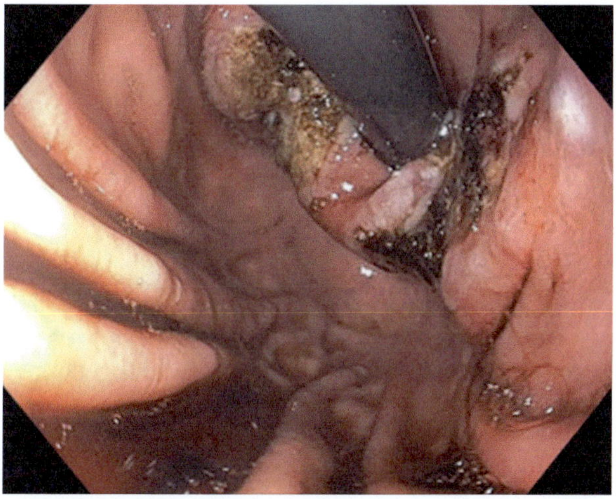

Fig. 2 Anti-reflux Mucosal Ablation (ARMA). The ARMA procedure is performed in the same distribution as ARMS and is done using argon plasma coagulation. The width of the ablation is around 1.5 cm

Potential Pitfalls

Once again, it is imperative to avoid ablating the esophageal mucosa, which can lead to stricture. When performing ARMA, the APC probe should not be in direct contact with the tissue, but rather, the probe should be slightly elevated from the tissue to allow for the appropriate arcing of current. If the probe is held in the same place for too long, then there is the potential for perforation. It is best practice to move the probe in a continuous and steady manner to avoid this problem.

Outcomes

The ARMA procedure was also pioneered by Inoue and was first reported in 2020 [35]. In their pilot study of 12 patients, Inoue et al. found a significant reduction in DeMeester Score (33.5 to 2.8) and improvement in GERD Health-Related Quality of Life (HRQL) at 2 months. Importantly, there were no complications reported. Since that time, ARMA has increased in popularity and there have been a number of systematic reviews comparing the outcomes between ARMS and ARMA [32, 36, 37]. Overall, the rates of symptomatic improvement for ARMS and ARMA are both above 80%. The most recent systematic review of ARMS vs ARMA actually notes a slightly higher rate of short-term success in the ARMA group at 88.3% [37]. The rate of perforation has also been noted to be higher for ARMS (2.2%) with no reported ARMA perforations in the literature [36]. More long-term data is needed to adequately assess the durability of these procedures and compare their outcomes to ARS.

Radiofrequency Ablation (RFA)

Technique and Key Steps

RFA is performed using the Stretta device (Restech Corporation, Houston, Texas, US), which is the only commercially available device for administering RFA for GERD. Stretta utilizes ablation of the distal esophagus induce tissue remodelling, decreased tissue compliance, and increased LES pressure [38]. Formal motility testing is also required prior to RFA as a major motility disorder is a contraindication. A hiatal hernia larger than 2 cm is also a contraindication.

A standard single channel endoscope is used for the procedure. During the initial assessment, measurements are taken to confirm the location GEJ. A guidewire is passed through the working channel of the endoscope and into the pylorus. The Stretta catheter is then thread over the wire towards the GEJ. The catheter has a balloon-basket assembly and nickel-titanium electrodes that apply RFA to the esophageal wall. Ablation is applied in six-locations ranging from 2 cm above to 2 cm below the Z-line. There are multiple treatments administered at each of the sites. After RFA is complete, endoscopy is again performed to rule out esophageal injury. In these patients, a PPI is continued in the immediate postoperative period and an esophageal diet is often prescribed to patients. This therapy can be offered to patients who have previously undergone ARS or bariatric surgery [39].

Potential Pitfalls

RFA is a safe and straightforward procedure to perform. Like other procedures where wires are used (e.g, dilations), it is important that the wire does not retract proximally when removing the endoscope. If this occurs and then the catheter is passed over the wire, it may increase the risk of perforation. Getting the correct measurements at the start of the procedure allows the endoscopist to ensure that they are ablating the correct areas. If this does not occur, then there is a chance that the desired areas will not be precisely ablated.

Outcomes

Early studies showed promising treatment results for RFA. Torquati et al. published one of the first series' on RFA and demonstrated a 3.3% reduction in AET [40]. Just over half of patients were able to completely wean from PPIs and 83% were highly satisfied with the procedure. Long-term cohort studies have shown continued efficacy up to a decade post-procedure [41, 42]. In the study by Noar et al., 41% of patients remained off of PPIs completely at 10 years and with 54% patient satisfaction. Notably, 85% of patients who had pre-existing BE had regression of disease on subsequent biopsies. Results from meta-analyses have been mixed. Fass et al. reviewed 28 prospective studies and found that RFA reduced esophageal acid exposure by 3%, halved the number of patients who required PPIs and improved GERD HRQL [43]. However, another meta-analysis compared Stretta to sham treatment and did not significant difference in GERD outcomes or GERD HRQL [44]. Overall, the data is less clearly defined for RFA in comparison to the other endoscopic therapies.

Conclusions and Future Direction

Endoscopic therapies for GERD provide promising treatment options for correctly selected patients. Although more long-term data is needed, present studies show superiority of TIF/ARMS/ARMA compared to PPI and sham while data for RFA is less clear. The main limitation of endoscopic therapies for GERD is the inability to address a large hiatal or paraesophageal hernia. TIF is now being combined with minimally invasive hiatal hernia repair in these instances; however, there are no studies directly comparing cTIF to ARS. Future studies should assess these outcomes and also examine the durability of each of these treatment options. As these procedures are generally safe and well-tolerated, they may become very useful in patients who are otherwise high-risk for surgery. If, in the future, surgical predictive modelling can identify patients who are likely to develop GERD after procedures like per oral endoscopic myotomy or laparoscopic sleeve gastrectomy, endoscopic therapies may even be considered concomitantly. As endoscopic therapies become more pervasive, surgeons should make it a priority to learn these techniques so they can continue to offer all treatment options to patients.

Acknowledgements Dr. Ayuso and Dr. Ujiki were the sole contributors to the content in this chapter. There were no other collaborators who helped with the drafting or editing of this work.

Competing Interests Dr. Ayuso receives educational grant money from Boston Scientific. Dr. Ujiki is an advisory board member for Boston Scientific and Apollo, a consultant and speaker for WL Gore and Medtronic, and a consultant for Olympus.

Ethics Approval Not applicable

References

1. El-Serag HB, Sweet S, Winchester CC, Dent J. Update on the epidemiology of gastro-oesophageal reflux disease: a systematic review. Gut [Internet]. 2014 [cited 2025 Apr 5];63(6):871–80. Available from: https://gut.bmj.com/content/63/6/871.
2. Sadafi S, Azizi A, Pasdar Y, Shakiba E, Darbandi M. Risk factors for gastroesophageal reflux disease: a population-based study. BMC Gastroenterol [Internet]. 2024 [cited 2025 Apr 5];24(1):64. Available from: https://pmc.ncbi.nlm.nih.gov/articles/PMC10840240/.
3. Dunn CP, Wu J, Gallagher SP, Putnam LR, Bildzukewicz NA, Lipham JC. Understanding the GERD barrier. J Clin Gastroenterol [Internet]. 2021 [cited 2025 Apr 5];55(6):459–68. Available from: https://pubmed.ncbi.nlm.nih.gov/33883513/.
4. Analatos A, Håkanson BS, Ansorge C, Lindblad M, Lundell L, Thorell A. Clinical outcomes of a laparoscopic total vs a 270° posterior partial fundoplication in chronic gastroesophageal reflux disease: a randomized clinical trial. JAMA Surg [Internet]. 2022 [cited 2025 Apr 5];157(6):473–80. Available from: https://jamanetwork.com/journals/jamasurgery/fullarticle/2791326.
5. Lafullarde T, Watson DI, Jamieson GG, Myers JC, Game PA, Devitt PG. Laparoscopic Nissen fundoplication: five-year results and beyond. Arch Surg [Internet]. 2001 [cited 2025 Apr 5];136(2):180–4. Available from: https://jamanetwork.com/journals/jamasurgery/fullarticle/390920.
6. Spechler SJ. The durability of antireflux surgery. JAMA [Internet]. 2017 [cited 2025 Apr 5];318(10):913–5. Available from: https://jamanetwork.com/journals/jama/fullarticle/2653718.
7. Nabi Z, Reddy DN. Endoscopic management of gastroesophageal reflux disease: revisited. Clin Endosc [Internet]. 2016 [cited 2025 Apr 5];49(5):408. Available from: https://pmc.ncbi.nlm.nih.gov/articles/PMC5066398/.
8. Chandra S, Gapp J, Wang K. Gastroesophageal reflux disorders: diagnostic approach. The AFS textbook of foregut disease [Internet]. 2023 [cited 2025 Apr 5];19–28. Available from: https://link.springer.com/chapter/10.1007/978-3-031-19671-3_3.
9. Lundell LR, Dent J, Bennett JR, Blum AL, Armstrong D, Galmiche JP, et al. Endoscopic assessment of oesophagitis: clinical and functional correlates and further validation of the Los Angeles classification. Gut [Internet]. 1999 [cited 2025 Apr 5];45(2):172–80. Available from: https://gut.bmj.com/content/45/2/172.

10. Hill LD, Kozarek RA, Kraemer SJM, Aye RW, Mercer CD, Low DE, et al. The gastroesophageal flap valve: in vitro and in vivo observations. Gastrointest Endosc. 1996;44(5):541–7.
11. Sharma P. Barrett esophagus: a review. JAMA [Internet]. 2022 [cited 2025 Apr 5];328(7):663–71. Available from: https://jamanetwork.com/journals/jama/fullarticle/2795263.
12. Bapaye J, Triadafilopoulos G, Iyer PG. Screening for Barrett's esophagus. The AFS textbook of foregut disease [Internet]. 2023 [cited 2025 Apr 5];147–59. Available from: https://mayoclinic.elsevierpure.com/en/publications/screening-for-barretts-esophagus-4.
13. Boeriu A, Boeriu C, Drasovean S, Pascarenco O, Mocan S, Stoian M, et al. Narrow-band imaging with magnifying endoscopy for the evaluation of gastrointestinal lesions. World J Gastrointest Endosc [Internet]. 2015 [cited 2025 Apr 5];7(2):110. Available from: https://pmc.ncbi.nlm.nih.gov/articles/PMC4325307/.
14. Qumseya B, Sultan S, Bain P, Jamil L, Jacobson B, Anandasabapathy S, et al. ASGE guideline on screening and surveillance of Barrett's esophagus Prepared by: ASGE STANDARDS OF PRACTICE COMMITTEE. Gastrointest Endosc [Internet]. 2019 [cited 2025 Apr 5];90(3). Available from: https://www.asge.org/docs/default-source/guidelines/asge-guideline-on-screening-and-surveillance-of-barrett-sesophagus-2019-september-gie.pdf.
15. Freedberg DE, Kim LS, Yang YX. The risks and benefits of long-term use of proton pump inhibitors: expert review and best practice advice from the American Gastroenterological Association. Gastroenterology. 2017;152(4):706–15.
16. Gyawali CP, Carlson DA, Chen JW, Patel A, Wong RJ, Yadlapati RH. ACG clinical guidelines: clinical use of esophageal physiologic testing. Am J Gastroenterol [Internet]. 2020 [cited 2025 Apr 5];115(9):1412–28. Available from: https://journals.lww.com/ajg/fulltext/2020/09000/acg_clinical_guidelines__clinical_use_of.19.aspx.
17. Richter JE, Pandolfino JE, Vela MF, Kahrilas PJ, Lacy BE, Ganz R, et al. Utilization of wireless pH monitoring technologies: a summary of the proceedings from the Esophageal Diagnostic Working Group. Dis Esophagus [Internet]. 2013 [cited 2025 Apr 5];26(8):755–65. Available from: https://doi.org/10.1111/j.1442-2050.2012.01384.x.
18. López-Alonso M, Moya MJ, Cabo JA, Ribas J, Macías MDC, Silny J, et al. Twenty-four-hour esophageal impedance-pH monitoring in healthy preterm neonates: rate and characteristics of acid, weakly acidic, and weakly alkaline gastroesophageal reflux. Pediatrics. 2006;118(2):e299–308.
19. Gyawali CP, Yadlapati R, Fass R, Katzka D, Pandolfino J, Savarino E, et al. Updates to the modern diagnosis of GERD: Lyon consensus 2.0. Gut [Internet]. 2024 [cited 2025 Apr 3];73(2):361–71. Available from: https://pubmed.ncbi.nlm.nih.gov/37734911/.
20. Amundson JR, Zukancic H, Kuchta K, Zimmermann CJ, VanDruff VN, Joseph S, et al. Acid exposure time better predicts outcomes following anti-reflux surgery than DeMeester score. Surg Endosc [Internet]. 2023 [cited 2025 Apr 5];37(8):6577–87. Available from: https://pubmed.ncbi.nlm.nih.gov/37311888/.
21. Yadlapati R, Gyawali CP, Pandolfino JE, Chang K, Kahrilas PJ, Katz PO, et al. AGA clinical practice update on the personalized approach to the evaluation and management of GERD: expert review. Clin Gastroenterol Hepatol [Internet]. 2022 [cited 2025 Apr 5];20(5):984–94.e1. Available from: https://pubmed.ncbi.nlm.nih.gov/35123084/.
22. Kondo T, Miwa H. The role of esophageal hypersensitivity in functional heartburn. J Clin Gastroenterol [Internet]. 2017 [cited 2025 Apr 7];51(7):571–8. Available from: https://journals.lww.com/jcge/fulltext/2017/08000/the_role_of_esophageal_hypersensitivity_in.3.aspx.
23. Ihde GM. The evolution of TIF: transoral incisionless fundoplication. Therap Adv Gastroenterol [Internet]. 2020 [cited 2025 Apr 7];13. Available from: https://journals.sagepub.com/doi/full/10.1177/1756284820924206.
24. Brewer Gutierrez OI, Choi D, Hejazi R, Samo S, Tran MN, Chang KJ, et al. American Foregut Society White Paper on transoral incisionless fundoplication. Foregut [Internet]. 2023 [cited 2025 Apr 7];3(3):242–54. Available from: https://journals-sagepub-com.libproxy.lib.unc.edu/doi/full/10.1177/26345161231170788?utm_source=summon&utm_medium=discovery-provider.

25. Jaber F, Ayyad M, Ayoub F, Patel KK, Makris KI, Hernaez R, et al. Concomitant hiatal hernia repair with transoral incisionless fundoplication for the treatment of refractory gastroesophageal reflux disease: a systematic review. Surg Endosc [Internet]. 2024 [cited 2025 Apr 7];38(10):5528–40. Available from: https://link.springer.com/article/10.1007/s00464-024-11201-2.
26. Trad KS, Barnes WE, Prevou ER, Simoni G, Steffen JA, Shughoury AB, et al. The TEMPO Trial at 5 years: transoral fundoplication (TIF 2.0) is safe, durable, and cost-effective. Surg Innov [Internet]. 2018 [cited 2025 Apr 7];25(2):149–57. Available from: https://pubmed.ncbi.nlm.nih.gov/29405886/.
27. Richter JE, Kumar A, Lipka S, Miladinovic B, Velanovich V. Efficacy of laparoscopic Nissen fundoplication vs transoral incisionless fundoplication or proton pump inhibitors in patients with gastroesophageal reflux disease: a systematic review and network meta-analysis. Gastroenterology. 2018;154(5):1298–308.e7.
28. Wu H, Ungerleider S, Attaar M, Wong HJ, Kuchta K, Denham W, et al. Tailored fundoplication for GERD with impedance planimetry (EndoFLIPTM). Foregut [Internet]. 2022 [cited 2025 Apr 7];2(3):242–52. Available from: https://journals.sagepub.com/doi/abs/10.1177/26345161221094841.
29. Hedberg HM, Kuchta K, Ujiki MB. First experience with banded anti-reflux mucosectomy (ARMS) for GERD: feasibility, safety, and technique (with video). J Gastrointest Surg [Internet]. 2019 [cited 2025 Apr 3];23(6):1274–8. Available from: https://pubmed.ncbi.nlm.nih.gov/30734179/.
30. Gao SJ, Zhu Z, Zhang L, Yin J, Ni XF, Chen L. A novel modified endoscopic method for treating patients with refractory gastro-esophageal disease and moderate hiatus hernia. Rev Esp Enferm Dig [Internet]. 2023 [cited 2025 Apr 7];115(9):496–503. Available from: http://www.ncbi.nlm.nih.gov/pubmed/37073697.
31. Sumi K, Inoue H, Kobayashi Y, Iwaya Y, Abad MRA, Fujiyoshi Y, et al. Endoscopic treatment of proton pump inhibitor-refractory gastroesophageal reflux disease with anti-reflux mucosectomy: experience of 109 cases. Dig Endosc [Internet]. 2021 [cited 2025 Apr 7];33(3):347–54. Available from: https://onlinelibrary.wiley.com/doi/full/10.1111/den.13727.
32. Rajat Garg A, Mohammed A, Singh A, Schleicher M, Thota PN, Rustagi T, et al. Anti-reflux mucosectomy for refractory gastroesophageal reflux disease: a systematic review and meta-analysis. Endosc Int Open [Internet]. 2022 [cited 2025 Apr 7];10(06):E854–64. Available from: http://www.thieme-connect.com/products/ejournals/html/10.1055/a-1802-0220.
33. Wong HJ, Su B, Attaar M, Kuchta K, Stearns S, Linn JG, et al. Anti-reflux mucosectomy (ARMS) results in improved recovery and similar reflux quality of life outcomes compared to laparoscopic Nissen fundoplication. Surg Endosc [Internet]. 2021 [cited 2025 Apr 7];35(12):7174–82. Available from: https://link.springer.com/article/10.1007/s00464-020-08144-9.
34. Callahan ZM, Amundson J, Su B, Kuchta K, Ujiki M. Outcomes after anti-reflux procedures: Nissen, Toupet, magnetic sphincter augmentation or anti-reflux mucosectomy? Surg Endosc [Internet]. 2023 [cited 2025 Apr 7];37(5):3944–51. Available from: https://pubmed.ncbi.nlm.nih.gov/35999311/.
35. Inoue H, Tanabe M, de Santiago ER, Abad MRA, Shimamura Y, Fujiyoshi Y, et al. Anti-reflux mucosal ablation (ARMA) as a new treatment for gastroesophageal reflux refractory to proton pump inhibitors: a pilot study. Endosc Int Open [Internet]. 2020 [cited 2025 Apr 7];8(2):E133. Available from: https://pmc.ncbi.nlm.nih.gov/articles/PMC6976329/.
36. Yeh JH, Lee CT, Hsu MH, Lin CW, Hsiao PJ, Chen CL, et al. Antireflux mucosal intervention (ARMI) procedures for refractory gastroesophageal reflux disease: a systematic review and meta-analysis. Therap Adv Gastroenterol [Internet]. 2022 [cited 2025 Apr 7];15. Available from: https://journals.sagepub.com/doi/full/10.1177/17562848221094959.
37. Al-Obaidi H, Merza N, Saab O, Al-Obaidi M, Agha I, Wakil A. S705 The efficacy of anti-reflux mucosectomy (ARMS) and antireflux mucosal ablation (ARMA) for gastroesophageal reflux disease (GERD) by 24-hour pH monitoring: systematic review and meta-analysis. Am J Gastroenterol [Internet]. 2024 [cited 2025 Apr 7];119(10S):S490. Available from: https://

journals.lww.com/ajg/fulltext/2024/10001/s705_the_efficacy_of_antireflux_mucosectomy__arms_.706.aspx.

38. Franciosa M, Triadafilopoulos G, Mashimo H. Stretta radiofrequency treatment for GERD: a safe and effective modality. Gastroenterol Res Pract [Internet]. 2013 [cited 2025 Apr 7];2013(1):783815. Available from: https://onlinelibrary.wiley.com/doi/full/10.1155/2013/783815.
39. Oh JS, Wright AS. Evaluation and management of patients with gastroesophageal reflux disease (GERD): radiofrequency ablation (RFA). The SAGES manual of flexible endoscopy [Internet]. 2020 [cited 2025 Apr 7];475–86. Available from: https://link.springer.com/chapter/10.1007/978-3-030-23590-1_24.
40. Torquati A, Houston HL, Kaiser J, Holzman MD, Richards WO. Long-term follow-up study of the Stretta procedure for the treatment of gastroesophageal reflux disease. Surg Endosc Other Interv Tech [Internet]. 2004 [cited 2025 Apr 7];18(10):1475–9. Available from: https://link.springer.com/article/10.1007/s00464-003-9181-y.
41. Noar M, Squires P, Noar E, Lee M. Long-term maintenance effect of radiofrequency energy delivery for refractory GERD: a decade later. Surg Endosc [Internet]. 2014 [cited 2025 Apr 7];28(8):2323–33. Available from: https://pubmed.ncbi.nlm.nih.gov/24562599/.
42. Kim SE. Long-term efficacy of endoscopic radiofrequency Stretta therapy for patients with refractory gastroesophageal reflux disease. Clin Endosc [Internet]. 2024 [cited 2025 Apr 7];57(1):48. Available from: https://pmc.ncbi.nlm.nih.gov/articles/PMC10834285/.
43. Fass R, Cahn F, Scotti DJ, Gregory DA. Systematic review and meta-analysis of controlled and prospective cohort efficacy studies of endoscopic radiofrequency for treatment of gastroesophageal reflux disease. Surg Endosc [Internet]. 2017 [cited 2025 Apr 7];31(12):4865–82. Available from: https://pubmed.ncbi.nlm.nih.gov/28233093/.
44. Lipka S, Kumar A, Richter JE. No evidence for efficacy of radiofrequency ablation for treatment of gastroesophageal reflux disease: a systematic review and meta-analysis. Clin Gastroenterol Hepatol. 2015;13(6):1058–67.e1.

Complications of Gastroesophageal Reflux Disease

Sofia Bertona, Francisco Schlottmann,
Fernando A. M. Herbella, and Marco G. Patti

Introduction

Gastroesophageal reflux disease (GERD) is a condition resulting from reflux of stomach contents into the esophagus causing troublesome symptoms and/or complications. Approximately 20% of the U.S. adult population is affected by GERD, and its prevalence has been rising over the years, mostly due to the epidemic of obesity [1].

Typical symptoms of GERD include heartburn, regurgitation, and dysphagia. However, patients can be affected by a broad spectrum of symptoms such as cough, wheezing, asthma, chest pain, hoarseness, among others. While lifestyle modifications and medical therapy (i.e., proton pump inhibitors) are effective in most patients, chronic GERD can lead to a range of serious complications as follows: erosive esophagitis, esophageal strictures, Barrett's esophagus and esophageal adenocarcinoma [2]. In addition, chronic microaspirations in patients with GERD can cause chronic and progressive lung diseases such as Idiopathic Pulmonary Fibrosis (IPF). Furthermore, GERD plays a key role in development of bronchiolitis obliterans syndrome (BOS), a main cause of lung transplant rejection.

S. Bertona (✉)
Department of Surgery, Hospital Alemán of Buenos Aires, Buenos Aires, Argentina
e-mail: sbertona@hospitalaleman.com

F. Schlottmann
University of Buenos Aires, Ciudad Autónoma Buenos Aires, Buenos Aires, Argentina

F. A. M. Herbella
Department of Surgery, Federal University of São Paulo, São Paulo, São Paulo, Brazil
e-mail: herbella.dcir@epm.br

M. G. Patti
Department of Surgery, University of Virginia Hospital, Charlottesville, VA, USA

F. Schlottmann et al. (eds.), *Esophageal Disorders*,
https://doi.org/10.1007/978-3-032-08179-7_6

Erosive Esophagitis

Erosive esophagitis is a severe form of esophageal mucosal inflammation that results from persistent reflux of gastric contents into the esophagus causing breaks, disruption and erosion of the mucosal cell layer [3, 4]. Esophagitis is one of the most common complications of GERD and is characterized by the endoscopic presence of ulcerations, erosions, and/or bleeding. While GERD is the most common cause of esophagitis, it is relevant to know that other potential factors (e.g. immune-related, medications, food) can also be involved [5].

The Los Angeles (LA) classification is a widespread method to determine the presence and severity of erosive esophagitis (Table 1). This classification system is based on findings from endoscopic examination of the esophagus. LA grade A refers to one or more mucosal breaks no longer than 5 mm, not bridging the tops of two mucosal folds. LA grade B refers to one or more mucosal breaks more than 5 mm long, not extending between the tops of two mucosal folds. LA grade C is defined by one or more mucosal breaks bridging the tops of mucosal folds involving less than 75% of the circumference. LA grade D is defined by one or more mucosal breaks bridging the tops of mucosal folds involving more than 75% of the circumference (Figs. 1 and 2).

The endoscopic assessment of esophagitis is associated with a high interobserver variability, especially for patients with low-grade esophagitis (LA A and LA B) [6]. While the presence of LA grade A is somehow non-specific and can be found in asymptomatic controls, Los Angeles grade C or D, Barrett's esophagus, or peptic strictures and currently considered confirmatory evidence for GERD [7–9].

Erosive esophagitis is detected in around 30% of treatment-naïve patients with heartburn and in less than 10% of patients receiving medical therapy. Therefore, non-erosive reflux disease (NERD) still represents the most frequent phenotypic presentation of GERD and includes patients who have typical symptoms without any mucosal breaks at endoscopy [10, 11].

Table 1 Los Angeles classification of esophagitis

Los Angeles classification of esophagitis	
Grade A	Mucosal breaks ≤5 mm long, none of which extends between the tops of the mucosal folds
Grade B	Mucosal breaks >5 mm long, none of which extends between the tops of two mucosal folds
Grade C	Mucosal breaks that extend between the tops of ≥2 mucosal folds, but which involve <75% of the esophageal circumference
Grade D	Mucosal breaks which involve ≥75% of the esophageal circumference

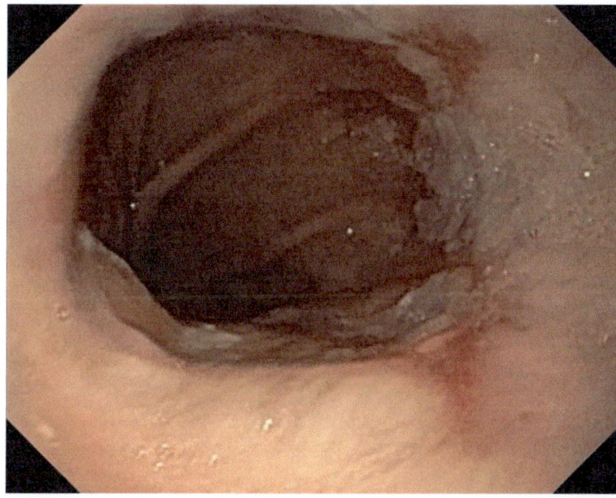

Fig. 1 Esophagitis Los Angeles grade B

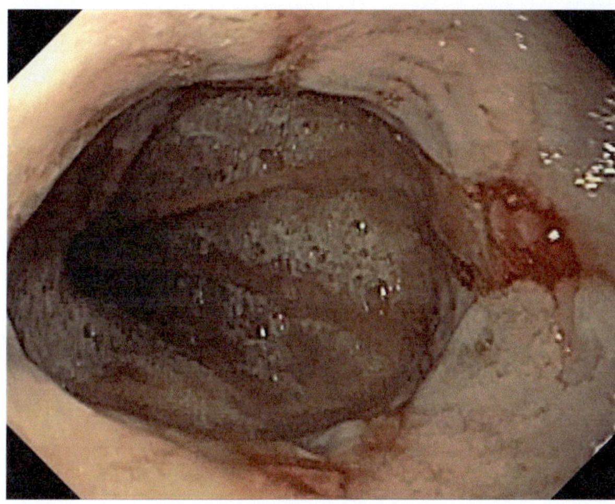

Fig. 2 Esophagitis Los Angeles grade C

Barrett's Esophagus

Barrett's esophagus (BE) is defined as the presence of at least 1 cm of metaplastic columnar epithelium replacing the stratified squamous epithelium normally lining the distal esophagus. The presence of intestinal metaplasia (columnar epithelium with goblet cells) is currently also required for the diagnosis of BE. The histopathological progression of BE extends from metaplasia to dysplasia and has the potential to advance to adenocarcinoma in the absence of treatment. Approximately 10–15% of the patients with GERD will ultimately develop BE, which is consider the main risk factor for esophageal adenocarcinoma [12].

Risk factors associated with the development of BE include frequent GERD symptoms, alcohol use, tobacco smoking, male gender, and obesity [13]. The presence of a large hiatal hernia is also associated with an increased risk of BE [14]. Based on patients' risk factors, the European Society of Gastrointestinal Endoscopy (ESGE) guidelines suggest screening for BE in patients ≥50 years of age with a history of chronic GERD symptoms, and at least one of the following risk factors: white ethnicity, male sex, obesity, smoking, and those having a first-degree relative with BE or esophageal adenocarcinoma [15].

A segment of BE measuring <3 cm is defined as short-segment BE, while a segment ≥3 cm is defined as long-segment BE. The Prague classification is recommended to provide a standardized description of BE. The classification measures the circumferential extent of metaplasia (C) and the maximal extent of metaplasia (M) [16] (Figs. 3 and 4).

The presumptive endoscopic diagnosis of BE should always be confirmed by the pathologist. Histologically, patients with BE are stratified as those with no dysplasia, indefinite for dysplasia, low-grade dysplasia (LGD), and high-grade dysplasia (HGD). Patients with no dysplasia and LGD have a significantly lower risk of progressing to esophageal adenocarcinoma (EAC) as compared to those with HGD [17, 18].

According to the American College of Gastroenterology [12], the management of BE is primarily guided by the presence of dysplasia. For patients with BE without dysplasia, repeat endoscopic surveillance is recommended every 3–5 years, depending on the length of the BE segment. In cases where BE is classified as indefinite for dysplasia, endoscopy should be repeated after 3–6 months, following optimization with acid suppression therapy. For BE with LGD, patients can either undergo endoscopic therapy with radiofrequency ablation or endoscopic surveillance every 12 months. Patients with HGD should always be treated endoscopically, unless life-limiting comorbidities are present.

The most commonly used endoscopic therapy for BE is radiofrequency ablation (RFA), which uses thermal energy to precisely remove damaged mucosal tissue. Adverse events such as strictures, bleeding, and perforation might occur [19].

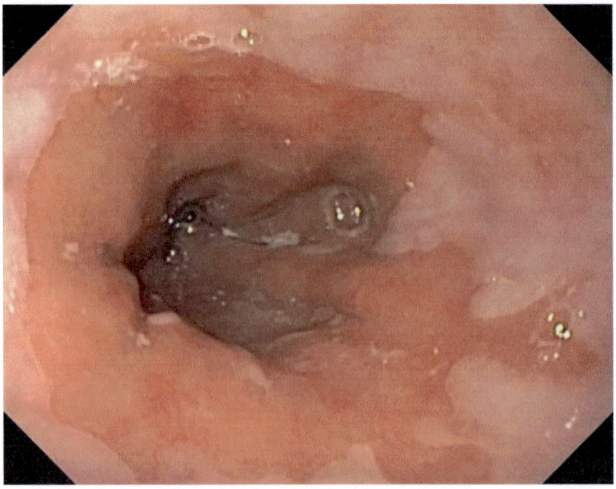

Fig. 3 Endoscopic image of a patient with Barrett's esophagus. Salmon-colored mucosa replaces the normal white pale mucosa lining the distal esophagus

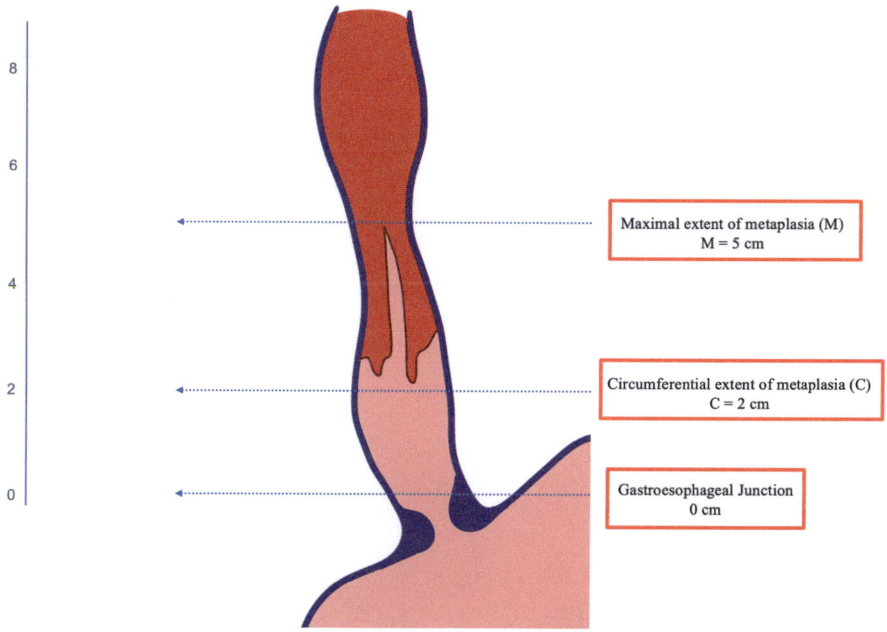

Fig. 4 Prague Classification for Barrett's esophagus. In this case, classified as C2 M5

Cryoablation can also be used, which consists in employing freezing and thawing to damage tissue, leading to necrosis. Unlike RFA, it does not alter the esophageal architecture and is less likely to cause strictures [20].

Esophageal Adenocarcinoma

Although only around 14% of all esophageal cancers are esophageal adenocarcinomas (EAC), it is the dominant subtype in Western Europe and North America. Over the past 40 years, the incidence of EAC has increased more than six-fold in Western countries (Fig. 5).

The increased incidence of EAC has been mostly related to the rising prevalence of obesity and GERD (and thereby BE). BE is a premalignant mucosa with increased proliferation rates and decreased apoptosis rates compared to normal epithelium. Although BE is the only known precursor of EAC, a relatively small percentage of patients with BE will eventually develop cancer and most patients with diagnosis of EAC have no prior history of BE. The question as to why some patients with BE progress to EAC and others do not remains unanswered [21, 22] (Fig. 6).

Patients with intramucosal carcinoma (T1a) are suitable for endoscopic therapies, such as endoscopic mucosal resection (EMR). Once a complete resection of the T1a adenocarcinoma is performed, the entire segment of BE should be treated

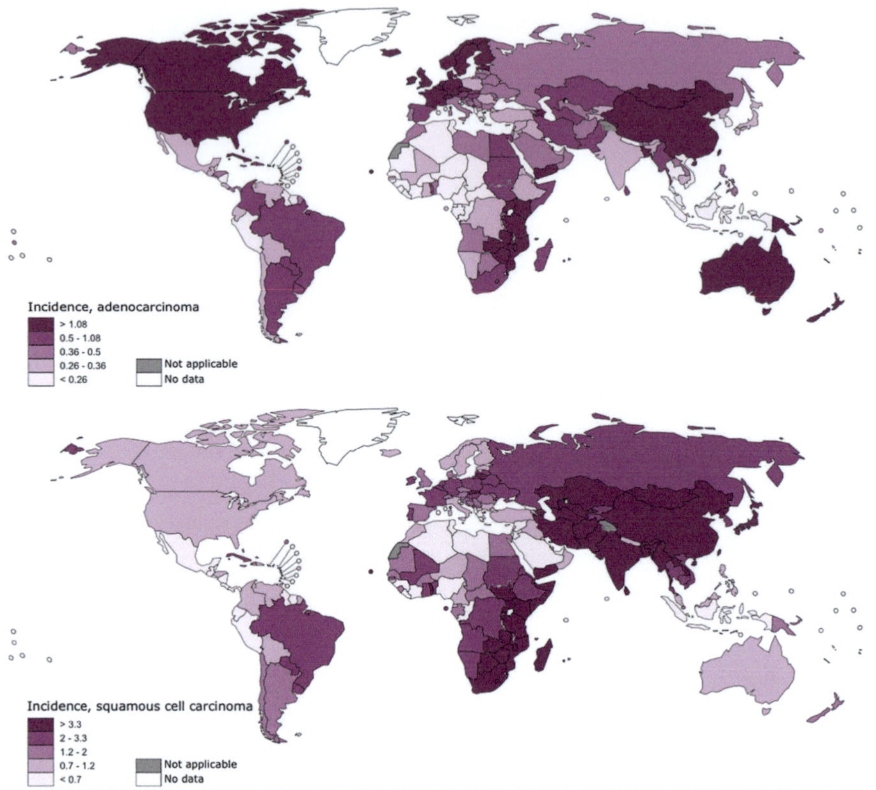

Fig. 5 Epidemiology of esophageal cancer. (Obtained with permission from the International Agency for Research on Cancer/World Health Organization (IARC/WHO)

with RFA. Previous research has shown that EMR successfully eradicates both EAC and BE in 98.8% of patients [23]. Combination therapy using EMR and RFA is associated to a lower risk of dysplasia recurrence and consequently development of EAC. As recurrence risk seems to be highest within the first 2 years post complete remission of intestinal metaplasia [24], this period requires close endoscopic follow-up. The most common complication of endoscopic resection is stricture followed by bleeding and perforation.

For selected patients with submucosal cancer (T1b), endoscopic therapy with endoscopic submucosal dissection (ESD) may be an alternative strategy to esophagectomy, especially in those with superficial (sm1) disease and well-differentiated neoplasm lacking lymphovascular invasion. Patients with deeper T1b tumors (sm2–sm3) or with high-risk pathological features (i.e., ulceration, poorly differentiated, lymphovascular invasion) should undergo esophagectomy.

Figure 7 shows an algorithm for the management of BE and early-stage EAC.

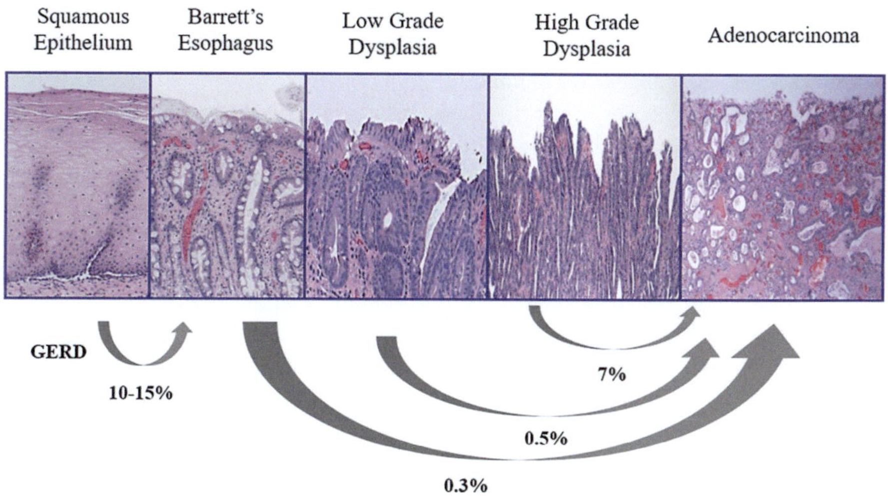

Fig. 6 Pathological progression from normal esophageal squamous epithelium to esophageal adenocarcinoma (From Esophageal Cancer: Diagnosis and Treatment 2nd edition. Editors Francisco Schlottmann, Lorenzo Ferri, Daniela Molena, Marco G Patti. Spinger 2023)

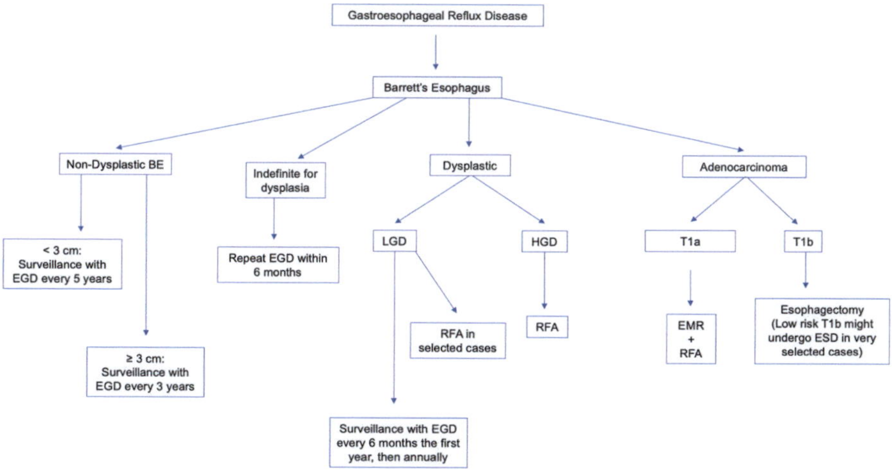

Fig. 7 Algorithm for the management of Barrett's esophagus and esophageal adenocarcinoma (EGD: esophagogastroduodenoscopy, LGD: low-grade dysplasia; HGD: high-grade dysplasia; RFA: radiofrequency ablation; EMR: endoscopic mucosal resection; ESD: endoscopic submucosal disection)

Esophageal Strictures

Esophageal strictures due to GERD represent the most frequent cause of benign esophageal strictures. Around 7–23% of patients with untreated GERD will develop an esophageal stricture [25, 26]. Acid reflux generates mucosal inflammation, which is initially reversible. As the esophageal exposure to acid reflux persists, inflammation progresses causing erosions and ulcerations, which leads to fibrosis and ultimately esophageal wall thickening and luminal constriction.

Strictures usually occur in the distal esophagus and typically tend to be 2–4 cm long. Schatzki rings are fibrous rings most commonly located in the lower esophagus which are also strongly associated with pathologic acid exposure. Although patients with GERD-related strictures typically present with dysphagia and weight loss, other GERD symptoms such as heartburn and regurgitation can exist. Medical therapy should be maximized to control esophageal inflammation and multiple biopsies of the stricture are recommended to rule out malignancy.

Endoscopic dilatations with either a bougie or balloon can be used in patients who do not respond to medication. It is recommended to start with small dilatation diameters (10 mm) and increase gradually over further procedures to reduce the risk of complications (i.e., perforation or bleeding). Endoscopic injection of steroids (e.g. triamcinolone) following dilatation can also be beneficial.

Pulmonary Complications

GERD can lead to extraesophageal symptoms related to the upper respiratory tract including chronic cough, hoarseness, and throat clearing. Many studies have shown a strong association between GERD and various respiratory conditions such as asthma, chronic obstructive pulmonary disease (COPD), chronic cough, and interstitial lung disease [27–29].

Asthma, COPD and Chronic Cough

The prevalence of GERD in patients with asthma ranges from 30 –90% [27]. Although the exact mechanism on how GERD and asthma are related is unclear, there are two main theories. The "***Reflux theory***" suggests that microaspiration of gastric contents damages the lungs, leading to cough, acute lung injury or even acute respiratory distress syndrome. This injury can result from airway obstruction, non-infectious chemical pneumonitis, or severe inflammatory responses like hypoxemia. The "***Reflex theory***" proposes an indirect mechanism in which distal esophageal acid reflux stimulates the vagal nerve, leading to bronchoconstriction. The effect of GERD on asthma exacerbation is still debatable because while some studies have shown positive results, others have demonstrated no clear effects on asthma outcomes [30–33]. A recent study concluded that the presence of GERD was an independent risk factor associated with uncontrolled asthma in patients with severe asthma treated with biological therapies [34]. However, a previous meta-analysis showed that the use proton pump inhibitors (PPI) was not associated with significant improvement in morning peak expiratory flow in asthma patients with GERD [35]. Overall, current evidence does not support PPI therapy as an empirical treatment in these patients.

COPD is a chronic, progressive condition, characterized by an increased inflammatory response within the airways and airflow limitation that is not fully reversible. The prevalence of GERD in individuals with COPD ranges from 17% to 54% [36]. Similar to asthma, micro-aspiration of gastric contents or bronchospasm induced by stimulation of the vagal nerve due to the irritation of the esophagus might contribute to the association between GERD and COPD. The presence of pathologic gastroesophageal reflux appears to be associated with increased pulmonary symptoms, poorer quality of life, and increased frequency of COPD exacerbations [37]. However, there are contradictory results regarding the effects of PPI therapy on COPD patients. A previous randomized trial comparing conventional therapy against conventional therapy plus lansoprazole for 12 months found that the use of PPIs was associated with a significant decrease of COPD exacerbations [38]. Another study also showed significant improvements in COPD symptom index after 2 months of PPI therapy in COPD patients with evidence of laryngopharyngeal reflux [39]. On the other hand, Sanchez and colleagues [40] reported that although PPIs significantly decreased the upright RYAN score (severity of laryngopharyngeal reflux), this was not associated with lung function improvements.

GERD might also be responsible of chronic cough in patients with no clear diagnosis of a respiratory disease. In fact, a previous study showed that chronic cough was reduced by 47% during the day and by 80% during the night after anti-reflux surgery [41], demonstrating a causal relationship between gastroesophageal reflux and chronic cough. Other studies, however, found contradictory results regarding the benefits of medical therapy or anti-reflux surgery in patients with GERD and chronic cough [42–44]. Based on the current evidence, it is rationale to consider anti-reflux surgery only in patients with objective diagnosis of GERD (i.e. pH monitoring) and troublesome symptoms (regurgitation and cough) despite medical therapy.

Idiopathic Pulmonary Fibrosis

Idiopathic Pulmonary Fibrosis (IPF) accounts for approximately 50–60% of all idiopathic interstitial pneumonias and has been strongly associated with GERD. IPF patients have shown significantly higher esophageal acid exposure, reflux episodes, and proximal reflux compared to non-IPF patients [45]. These findings suggest that IPF patients are at high risk of aspiration of gastric contents, advocating the need for effective anti-reflux therapy.

Raghu et al reported that almost 90% of IPF patients have pathologic esophageal acid reflux, with 76% and 63% abnormal distal and proximal exposure, respectively [46]. Contributing factors to reflux in IPF include a hypotensive LES, abnormal esophageal peristalsis, presence of a hiatal hernia and increased transdiaphragmatic pressure gradient [47–50]. Anti-reflux surgery is an attractive alternative on these patients because a fundoplication restores the LES competence, controlling both acidic and non-acidic reflux. However, evidence on the efficacy of anti-reflux surgery in IPF patients is still weak and conflicting [51–54]. In fact, the American

Thoracic Society and other international societies recently published clinical practice guidelines for IPF and recommend against treating patients with PPIs or anti-reflux surgery for the sole purpose of improving respiratory outcomes [55].

Bronchiolitis Obliterans Syndrome

Lung transplantation is an available therapy for end-stage lung diseases like IPF. Unfortunately, the five-year survival rate post-transplant is around 50%, much lower than other organ transplants like heart (75%) or liver (70%). This low survival rate is mostly related to both acute and chronic rejection, with the latter manifesting as bronchiolitis obliterans syndrome (BOS), which is a progressive decline in the forced expiratory volume in 1s (FEV1).

GERD has also been recognized as a risk factor for the development of BOS through continuous aspiration of gastric contents. Bile acids and pepsin (a proteolytic enzyme) have been found in the bronchoalveolar lavage fluid of lung transplant patients. Aspiration of gastric contents ultimately impair the immunity of the transplanted lung [56, 57]. GERD affects around two-thirds of lung-transplant patients. Factors contributing to GERD include vagal nerve injury, delayed gastric emptying, immunosuppressive medications, and changes in intrathoracic and intra-abdominal pressures. Several studies have shown benefits of early anti-reflux surgery in preventing BOS and improving survival [58–60]. For this reason, it is currently recommended to routinely test for GERD in these patients, and strongly consider anti-reflux surgery before BOS develops.

Conclusions

A broad range of troublesome and sometimes life threating complications can occur in patients with GERD. Early diagnosis and adequate therapy are critical to prevent long-term disability and improve patient outcomes.

Conflict of Interest The authors have no conflicts of interest.

References

1. El-Serag HN, Sweet S, Winchester CC, et al. Update on the epidemiology of gastro-esophageal reflux disease: a systematic review. Gut. 2014;63(6):871–80.
2. Fisichella PM, Schlottmann F, Patti MG. Evaluation of gastroesophageal reflux disease. Updates Surg. 2018;70(3):309–13.
3. Adachi K, Fujishiro H, Katsube T, et al. Predominant nocturnal acid reflux in patients with Los Angeles grade C and D reflux esophagitis. J Gastroenterol Hepatol. 2001;16(11):1191–6.
4. McDougall NI, Johnston BT, Collins JS, et al. Disease progression in gastro-oesophageal reflux disease as determined by repeat oesophageal pH monitoring and endoscopy 3–4.5 years after diagnosis. Eur J Gastroenterol Hepatol. 1997;9(12):1161–7.

5. Grossi L, Ciccaglione AF, Marzio L. Esophagitis and its causes: who is "guilty" when acid is found "not guilty"? World J Gastroenterol. 2017;23:3011–6.
6. Nasseri-Moghaddam S, Razjouyan H, Nouraei M, et al. Inter- and intra-observer variability of the Los Angeles classification: a reassessment. Arch Iran Med. 2007;10(1):48–53. Erratum in: Arch Iran Med. 2007;10(3):429
7. Takashima T, Iwakiri R, Sakata Y, et al. Endoscopic reflux esophagitis and Helicobacter pylori infection in young healthy Japanese volunteers. Digestion. 2012;86(1):55–8.
8. Visaggi P, Del Corso G, Gyawali CP, et al. Ambulatory pH-impedance findings confirm that grade B esophagitis provides objective diagnosis of gastroesophageal reflux disease. Am J Gastroenterol. 2023;118:794–801.
9. Gyawali CP, Yadlapati R, Fass R, et al. Updates to the modern diagnosis of GERD: Lyon consensus 2.0. Gut. 2024;73:361–71.
10. Savarino E, Zentilin P, Savarino V. NERD: an umbrella term including heterogeneous subpopulations. Nat Rev Gastroenterol Hepatol. 2013;10(6):371–80.
11. Kwak YE, Saleh A, Abdelwahed A, et al. Effectiveness of esophagogastroduodenoscopy in changing treatment outcome in refractory gastro-esophageal reflux disease. Scand J Gastroenterol. 2022;57(1):124–30.
12. Shaheen NJ, Falk GW, Iyer PG, et al. American college of gastro-enterology. ACG clinical guideline: diagnosis and management of Barrett's esophagus. Am J Gastroenterol. 2016;111(1):30–50.
13. Antonios K, Aintabi D, McNally P, et al. Risk factors for the development of Barrett's esophagus and esophageal adenocarcinoma: a systematic review and meta-analysis. Cancer Rep (Hoboken). 2025;8(3):e70168.
14. Ma S, Tong Z, He Y, et al. Association between hiatal hernia and Barrett's esophagus: an updated meta-analysis with trial sequential analysis. Therap Adv Gastroenterol. 2024;17:17562848231219234.
15. Weusten BLAM, Bisschops R, Dinis-Ribeiro M, et al. Diagnosis and management of Barrett esophagus: European Society of Gastrointestinal Endoscopy (ESGE) Guideline. Endoscopy. 2023;55(12):1124–46.
16. Sharma P, Dent J, Armstrong D, et al. The development and validation of an endoscopic grading system for Barrett's esophagus: the Prague C & M criteria. Gastroenterology. 2006;131(5):1392–9.
17. Singh S, Manickam P, Amin AV, et al. Incidence of esophageal adenocarcinoma in Barrett's esophagus with low-grade dysplasia: a systematic review and meta-analysis. Gastrointest Endosc. 2014;79(6):897–909.e4. quiz 983.e1, 983.e3
18. Rastogi A, Puli S, El-Serag HB, et al. Incidence of esophageal adenocarcinoma in patients with Barrett's esophagus and high-grade dysplasia: a meta-analysis. Gastrointest Endosc. 2008;67(3):394–8.
19. Wang Y, Ma B, Yang S, et al. Efficacy and safety of radiofrequency ablation vs. endoscopic surveillance for Barrett's esophagus with low-grade dysplasia: meta-analysis of randomized controlled trials. Front Oncol. 2022;12:801940.
20. Papaefthymiou A, Norton B, Telese A, et al. Efficacy and safety of cryoablation in Barrett's esophagus and comparison with radiofrequency ablation: a meta-analysis. Cancers (Basel). 2024;16(17):2937.
21. Desai TK, Krishnan K, Samala N, et al. The incidence of oesophageal adenocarcinoma in non-dysplastic Barrett's oesophagus: a meta-analysis. Gut. 2012;61(7):970–6.
22. Corley DA, Mehtani K, Quesenberry C, et al. Impact of endoscopic surveillance on mortality from Barrett's esophagus-associated esophageal adenocarcinomas. Gastroenterology. 2013;145(2):312–9.e1.
23. Konda VJ, Gonzalez Haba Ruiz M, et al. Complete endoscopic mucosal resection is effective and durable treatment for Barrett's-associated neoplasia. Clin Gastroenterol Hepatol. 2014;12(12):2002–10.e1–2.
24. He T, Sundararajan V, Clark NJ, et al. Long-term outcomes after endoscopic eradication therapy for dysplastic and T1a adenocarcinoma related Barrett's esophagus: higher rate of

late dysplastic recurrence with radio-frequency ablation monotherapy. Gastrointest Endosc. 2025;S0016-5107(25):00050–1.
25. Xue AZ, Anderson C, Cotton CC, et al. Prevalence and costs of esophageal strictures in the United States. Clin Gastroenterol Hepatol. 2024;22(9):1821–1829.e4.
26. Richter JE. Peptic strictures of the esophagus. Gastroenterol Clin N Am. 1999;28(4):875–91.
27. Broers C, Tack J, Pauwels A. Review article: gastro-oesophageal reflux disease in asthma and chronic obstructive pulmonary disease. Aliment Pharmacol Ther. 2018;47(2):176–91.
28. Zhou JC, Gavini S, Chan WW, Lo WK. Relationship between esophageal disease and pulmonary fibrosis. Dig Dis Sci. 2023;68(4):1096–105.
29. Ruaro B, Pozzan R, Confalonieri P, Tavano S, Hughes M, Matucci Cerinic M, Baratella E, Zanatta E, Lerda S, Geri P, Confalonieri M, Salton F. Gastroesophageal reflux disease in idiopathic pulmonary fibrosis: viewer or actor? To treat or not to treat? Pharmaceuticals (Basel). 2022;15(8):1033.
30. ten Brinke A, Sterk PJ, Masclee AA, Spinhoven P, Schmidt JT, Zwinderman AH, Rabe KF, Bel EH. Risk factors of frequent exacerbations in difficult-to-treat asthma. Eur Respir J. 2005;26(5):812–8.
31. Cheung TK, Lam B, Lam KF, et al. Gastroesophageal reflux disease is associated with poor asthma control, quality of life, and psychological status in Chinese asthma patients. Chest. 2009;135(5):1181–5.
32. Liang B, Yi Q, Feng Y. Association of gastroesophageal reflux disease with asthma control. Dis Esophagus. 2013;26(8):794–8.
33. Iqbal N, Amirali A, Lail GU, Khan MA, Sial R, Irfan M. Correlation of gastro-esophageal reflux disease with asthma control and quality of life: a cross-sectional study from a low-middle income country. Ther Adv Respir Dis. 2024;18:17534666241297879.
34. Guilleminault L, Camus C, Raherison-Semjen C, et al. Improvement in severe asthma patients receiving biologics and factors associated with persistent insufficient control: a real-life national study. Ther Adv Respir Dis. 2023;17:17534666231202749.
35. Zheng Z, Luo Y, Li J, Gao J. Randomised trials of proton pump inhibitors for gastro-oesophageal reflux disease in patients with asthma: an updated systematic review and meta-analysis. BMJ Open. 2021;11(8):e043860.
36. Lee AL, Goldstein RS. Gastroesophageal reflux disease in COPD: links and risks. Int J Chron Obstruct Pulmon Dis. 2015;10:1935–49.
37. Huang C, Liu Y, Shi G. A systematic review with meta-analysis of gastroesophageal reflux disease and exacerbations of chronic obstructive pulmonary disease. BMC Pulm Med. 2020;20(1):2.
38. Sasaki T, Nakayama K, Yasuda H, et al. A randomized, single-blind study of lansoprazole for the prevention of exacerbations of chronic obstructive pulmonary disease in older patients. J Am Geriatr Soc. 2009;57(8):1453–7.
39. Eryuksel E, Dogan M, Olgun S, et al. Incidence and treatment results of laryngopharyngeal reflux in chronic obstructive pulmonary disease. Eur Arch Otorhinolaryngol. 2009;266(8):1267–71.
40. Sanchez J, Schumann DM, Karakioulaki M, et al. Laryngopharyngeal reflux in chronic obstructive pulmonary disease – a multi-centre study. Respir Res. 2020;21(1):220.
41. Ekström T, Johansson KE. Effects of anti-reflux surgery on chronic cough and asthma in patients with gastro-oesophageal reflux disease. Respir Med. 2000;94(12):1166–70.
42. Ribolsi M, Savarino E, De Bortoli N, et al. Reflux pattern and role of impedance-pH variables in predicting PPI response in patients with suspected GERD-related chronic cough. Aliment Pharmacol Ther. 2014;40(8):966–73.
43. Ours TM, Kavuru MS, Schilz RJ, Richter JE. A prospective evaluation of esophageal testing and a double-blind, randomized study of omeprazole in a diagnostic and therapeutic algorithm for chronic cough. Am J Gastroenterol. 1999;94(11):3131–8.
44. Chang AB, Lasserson TJ, Kiljander TO, et al. Systematic review and meta-analysis of randomised controlled trials of gastro-oesophageal reflux interventions for chronic cough associated with gastro-oesophageal reflux. BMJ. 2006;332(7532):11–7.

45. Savarino E, Carbone R, Marabotto E, et al. Gastro-oesophageal reflux and gastric aspiration in idiopathic pulmonary fibrosis patients. Eur Respir J. 2013;42(5):1322–31.
46. Raghu G, Freudenberger TD, Yang S, et al. High prevalence of abnormal acid gastro-oesophageal reflux in idiopathic pulmonary fibrosis. Eur Respir J. 2006;27(1):136–42.
47. Patti MG, Tedesco P, Golden J, et al. Idiopathic pulmonary fibrosis: how often is really idiopathic? J Gastrointest Surg. 2005;9:1053–8.
48. Sweet MP, Herbella FAM, Leard L, et al. The prevalence of distal and proximal gastroesophageal reflux in patients awaiting lung transplantation. Ann Surg. 2006;244:491–7.
49. Noth I, Zangan SM, Soares RV, et al. Prevalence of hiatal hernia by blinded multidetector CT in patients with idiopathic pulmonary fibrosis. Eur Respir J. 2012;39(2):344–51.
50. Del Grande LM, Herbella FAM, Patti MG. The role of the Transdiaphragmatic Pressure Gradient (TGP) in the pathophysiology of proximal reflux. J Gastrointest Surg. 2021;25(2):351–6.
51. Linden PA, Gilbert RJ, Yeap BY, et al. Laparoscopic fundoplication in patients with end-stage lung disease awaiting transplantation. J Thorac Cardiovasc Surg. 2006;131(2):438–46.
52. Hoppo T, Jarido V, Pennathur A, et al. Antireflux surgery preserves lung function in patients with gastroesophageal reflux disease and end-stage lung disease before and after lung transplantation. Arch Surg. 2011;146:1041–7.
53. Raghu G, Pellegrini CA, Yow E, et al. Laparoscopic anti-reflux surgery for the treatment of idiopathic pulmonary fibrosis (WRAP-IPF): a multicentre, randomized, controlled phase 2 trial. Lancet Respir Med. 2018;6:707–14.
54. Khor YH, Bissell B, Ghazipura M, et al. Antacid medication and antireflux surgery in patients with idiopathic pulmonary fibrosis: a systematic review and meta-analysis. Ann Am Thorac Soc. 2022;19(5):833–44.
55. Raghu G, Remy-Jardin M, Richeldi L, et al. Idiopathic pulmonary fibrosis (an update) and progressive pulmonary fibrosis in adults: an official ATS/ERS/JRS/ALAT clinical practice guideline. Am J Respir Crit Care Med. 2022;205(9):e18–47.
56. D'Ovidio F, Mura M, Tsang M, et al. Bile acid aspiration and the development of bronchiolitis obliterans after lung transplantation. J Thorac Cardiovasc Surg. 2005;129(5):1144–52.
57. Stovold R, Forrest IA, Corris PA, et al. Pepsin, a biomarker of gastric aspiration in lung allografts: a putative association with rejection. Am J Respir Crit Care Med. 2007;175:1298–303.
58. Davis RD, Lau CL, Messier RH, et al. Improved lung allograft function after fundoplication in patients with gastroesophageal reflux disease undergoing lung transplantation. J Thorac Cardiovasc Surg. 2003;125:533–42.
59. Cantu E, Appel JZ 3rd, Hartwig MG, et al. Early fundoplication prevents chronic allograft dysfunction in patients with gastroesophageal reflux disease. Ann Thorac Surg. 2004;78:1142–51.
60. Gasper WJ, Sweet MP, Hoopes C, et al. Antireflux surgery for patients with end-stage lung disease before and after lung transplantation. Surg Endosc. 2008;22:495–500.

Management of Failed Anti-reflux Surgery

Sofia Bertona, Marco G. Patti, Fernando A. M. Herbella, and Francisco Schlottmann

Introduction

Anti-reflux surgery (ARS) is a well-established therapy for patients with gastroesophageal reflux disease (GERD) who do not respond adequately to medication, achieving control of symptoms in about 80 to 90% of patients [1–3]. A proportion of patients, however, will eventually experience persistence or recurrence of GERD-related symptoms [4]. Management of patients who fail ARS is complex and requires a thorough evaluation.

Failure of ARS can be related to three main causes: poor surgeon judgement in patient selection, anatomical failure and/or physiologic failure. A successful anti-reflux operation indeed requires a patient who was appropriately selected for the procedure, with symptoms attributable to pathologic acid reflux. Anatomical failure refers to complications or inadequacies of the surgical procedure itself. Physiologic failure consists in the onset of gastrointestinal symptoms despite a technically successful surgery (Table 1).

Understanding the causes and mechanisms behind the failure of ARS is crucial for improving patient outcomes and minimizing complications.

S. Bertona (✉)
Department of Surgery, Hospital Alemán of Buenos Aires, Buenos Aires, Argentina
e-mail: sbertona@hospitalaleman.com

M. G. Patti
Department of Surgery, University of Virginia Hospital, Charlottesville, VA, USA

F. A. M. Herbella
Department of Surgery, Federal University of São Paulo, São Paulo, São Paulo, Brazil
e-mail: herbella.dcir@epm.br

F. Schlottmann
University of Buenos Aires, Ciudad Autónoma Buenos Aires, Buenos Aires, Argentina

F. Schlottmann et al. (eds.), *Esophageal Disorders*,
https://doi.org/10.1007/978-3-032-08179-7_7

Table 1 Causes of anti-reflux surgery failures

Judgement failures	Anatomical failures	Physiological failures
Incomplete work-up	Poorly constructed fundoplication	Dysphagia
Misdiagnosis (primary esophageal motility disorder)	Disrupted fundoplication	Gas-related symptoms
Misdiagnosis (other gastrointestinal disorder)	Slipped fundoplication	Gastroparesis
Poor choice of fundoplication	Herniated fundoplication	Accelerated gastric emptying
High perioperative risks	Paraesophageal herniation type II/II/IV	Diarrhea
Psycho-emotional variables that might affect outcomes		

Potential Mechanisms Related to Anti-reflux Surgery Failure

Poor Surgeon Judgement in Patient Selection

Indication for ARS results from an accurate and thorough diagnostic evaluation of patients with GERD symptoms. Heartburn, regurgitation, and dysphagia are considered typical symptoms of GERD. However, many patients affected by GERD can present with extraesophageal symptoms such as cough, wheezing, asthma, chest pain, hoarseness, and/or dental erosions [5]. A previous study found that when GERD is diagnosed only based on heartburn and regurgitation, approximately one-third of patients have normal esophageal acid exposure [6]. A complete preoperative workup should include clinical history (including the evaluation of the response to medical therapy), barium swallow, upper endoscopy, esophageal manometry, and ambulatory pH monitoring [7].

Frequent misdiagnoses include patient's symptoms not related to pathological acid reflux (e.g., functional heartburn or cholelithiasis) or presence of an underlying esophageal motility disorder (mainly achalasia). Previous research has shown that the three most important predictors of successful outcome after ARS are the presence of typical symptoms, adequate symptomatic response to PPI therapy, and pathologic gastroesophageal reflux determined by pH monitoring [8]. The esophageal manometry is important not only to rule out primary esophageal motility disorders, but could also help tailoring the operation, especially on whether to perform a total or partial fundoplication (i.e., partial fundoplication is preferred in patients with severe esophageal dysmotility) [9].

Anatomical Failures

Several anatomical failures can occur after ARS [10] (Fig. 1):

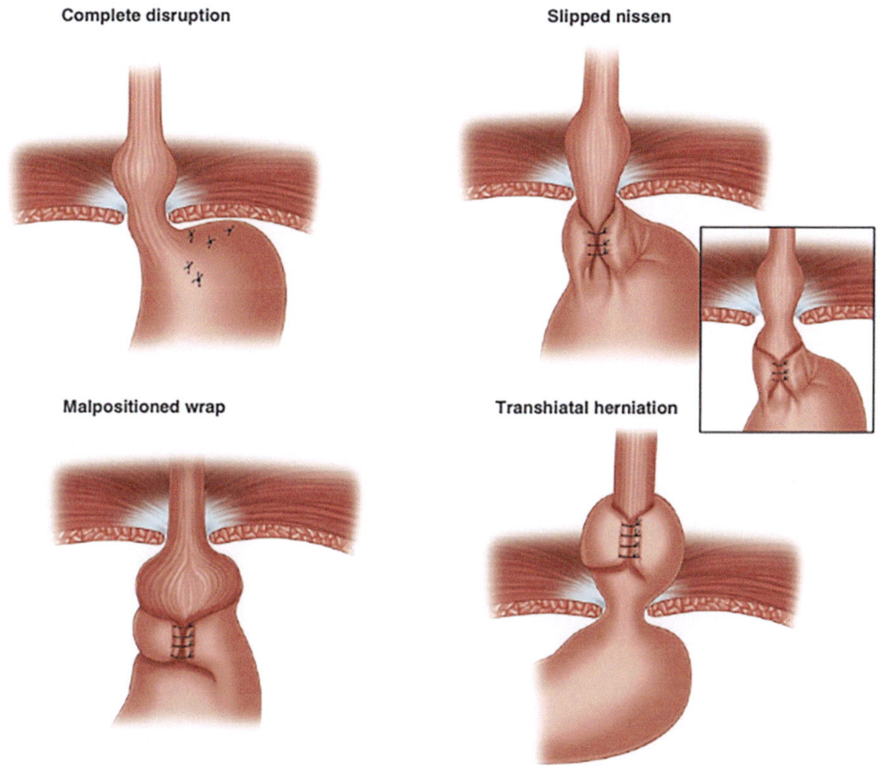

Fig. 1 Types of anatomical failures. (From foregut surgery: achalasia, gastroesophageal reflux disease and obesity. Editors Marco G. Patti, Marco Di Corpo, Francisco Schlottmann. Spinger 2020)

Poorly Constructed Fundoplication: The wrap should be located on the distal esophagus just superior to the esophagogastric junction (EGJ). A common "malpositioned" fundoplication is the one located around the stomach below the EGJ. Other technical errors include using the greater curvature of the stomach inferior to the fundus or twisting the vertical axis of the EGJ (ultimately kinking the esophagus and impairing adequate emptying into the stomach). A too tight fundoplication is another poorly constructed wrap. This can be related to insufficient section of short gastric vessels to allow for a floppy fundoplication. The use of a bougie/endoscope inside the esophagus can help avoiding this technical issue.

The poorly constructed wrap usually leads to persistent dysphagia, bloating, nausea, inability to belch, and/or inability to vomit.

Slipped Fundoplication: This occurs when the fundoplication, which was placed in the proper position above the EGJ, moves inferiorly so that the wrap ends encircling the proximal stomach or the proximal stomach moves superiorly through the fundoplication. Ultimately, a portion of the stomach is now located above the wrap and is herniated into the mediastinum. This issue often results from an excessively floppy wrap [11].

The slipped fundoplication can lead several symptoms including heartburn, dysphagia, upper abdominal pain, lower chest pain, and/or bloating.

Transhiatal Herniation of the Wrap: A "herniated" fundoplication occurs when both the EGJ and well-positioned intact wrap are herniated above the hiatus into the posterior mediastinum. This is commonly related to an inadequate closure of the hiatus. However, in some cases the hiatal opening can be enlarged due to progressive widening of the hiatus (with intact initial closure and sutures in place).

Persistent or recurrent heartburn or regurgitation are common symptoms in these patients. Dysphagia, bloating or upper abdominal pain can also occur.

Disrupted Fundoplication: A disrupted fundoplication occurs when the sutures holding the wrap in place break or become untied, which ultimately causes the wrap to lose its function as a competent sphincter. This can occur after episodes of increased intra-abdominal pressure causing tearing of suture (acute episode of retching or persistent cough). Patients will often complain of heartburn and regurgitation.

Paraesophageal Hernia with and Without Hernia Recurrence: In this case, a portion of the stomach, usually the greater curvature, or some other intra-abdominal organ herniates through the hiatus along alongside to the esophagus. It can be classified as follows: type II (EGJ and fundoplication still inferior to the hiatus in the abdomen), type III (EGJ with or without an intact fundoplication migrated into the posterior mediastinum), or type IV (with some intra-abdominal organ other that the stomach herniated into the mediastinum). When the hiatal repair remains intact, the likelihood of incarceration and strangulation of the herniated tissue increases significantly. Therefore, these patients can present with the same symptoms as the other anatomical failures with the added risk of incarceration or strangulation.

Previous studies have investigated the incidence and underlying causes of anatomical failures following ARS. One study found that approximately 7% of patients undergoing laparoscopic ARS experienced fundoplication failure, with most failures occurring during the surgeon's learning phase [12]. Furthermore, research on reoperative ARS for failed fundoplication revealed that transmediastinal migration of the wrap was the most common failure pattern observed [13].

Physiological Failures

Physiological failures of ARS are defined as alterations in the patient's physiology which leads to adverse symptomatic consequences. Unfortunately, the mechanisms are often not well understood.

Dysphagia: Early postoperative dysphagia is common and is often related to edema at the site of the fundoplication. Most patients are adequately managed with soft diet for a few weeks. Persistent dysphagia (>3–4 weeks) should alert of a possible anatomical failure previously discussed. Therefore, endoscopy and upper GI can be helpful to identify a technical issue. Dysphagia due to esophageal dysmotility should be considered when no anatomical failures are identified. The esophageal manometry can help for the diagnosis of an esophageal motility disorder (e.g. ineffective esophageal motility or achalasia either missed before ARS or developed postoperatively as a pseudo-achalasia pattern). A hypercontractile pattern can also occur in response to an obstruction after fundoplication.

Gas-Related Symptoms: Bloating, inability to belch, early satiety, and flatulence are symptoms that may occur after a fundoplication. The reasons why some patients experience these gas-related issues while others do not remain unclear. Potential contributing factors of the inability to vent gas from the stomach into the esophagus may be related to the impaired relaxation of the EGJ valve in response to gastric distension, aerophagia (which is relatively common among patients with severe GERD), and vagus nerve injury. The Nissen fundoplication (total 360°) is more commonly related to these symptoms than the partial fundoplication [4, 14]. Dietary modifications (such as avoiding gas-producing foods and carbonated beverages), slower eating to reduce aerophagia, and gas-reducing agents like simethicone can help managing gas-related symptoms. Prokinetic medications may also be beneficial [15].

Gastroparesis: Gastroparesis following ARS is relatively uncommon beyond the immediate postoperative period. Symptoms include nausea, vomiting, bloating and abdominal pain among others. When patients present with symptoms of gastroparesis post-fundoplication, it is crucial to determine whether these symptoms existed before the operation or developed after it. Gastroparesis can be idiopathic, diabetic, or related to an injury of the vagus nerve during ARS [15, 16]. Vagus nerve injury can occur if the nerve is not properly identified during the operation, particularly in cases involving large hiatal hernias or redo operations [17].

Diarrhea: Although postoperative diarrhea is relatively common after ARS, its pathophysiology is not yet fully understood. Possible contributing factors could be enhanced gastric emptying contributing to a more rapid gut transit, inadvertent vagotomy, changes in diet after the operation (e.g., liquid and soft diets) and/or exacerbation of underlying irritable bowel syndrome, among others. Antimotility drugs, antibiotics for small bowel overgrowth, and cholestyramine can be empirically used in these patients.

Evaluation of Patients with Persistent of Recurrent Symptoms

When assessing a patient with recurrent symptoms after ARS, it is crucial to conduct a thorough medical history, physical exam, and diagnostic work-up to accurately determine the cause of their symptoms. Key questions to ask include:

- Are the symptoms identical to those experienced before ARS?
- Was the patient adequately studied before ARS? (i.e. esophageal manometry and pH monitoring)
- Over what period of time have the symptoms returned?
- Is the patient on medication? Is there any symptomatic response to medical therapy?

Upper Endoscopy and Barium Swallow

Both tests are useful for evaluation of anatomical failures after fundoplication. Endoscopy helps assessing the presence and severity of esophagitis, presence of hiatal hernia, and integrity of the fundoplication valve. When evaluating the fundoplication in the retroflexed position, the gastric folds should be below the diaphragm, parallel to it. Abnormalities such as gastric folds above the diaphragm may indicate herniation or slippage of the stomach, while an absence of folds suggests total disruption of the wrap. (Fig. 2). Barium esophagram complements endoscopy by defining the EGJ anatomy, detecting hernias, and assessing esophageal emptying.

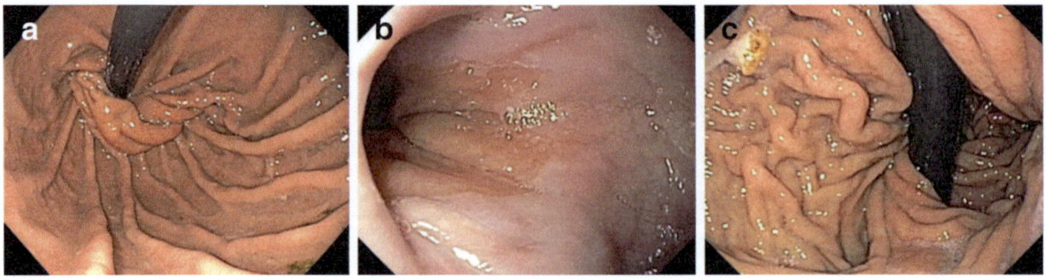

Fig. 2 Endoscopic views after a fundoplication. (**a**) Retroflexed view of an intact Nissen fundoplication. (**b**) Evidence of EGJ at 34 cm and hiatus at 41 cm, interpreted as a recurrent sliding hiatal hernia. (**c**) Disrupted fundoplication and recurrent hiatal hernia

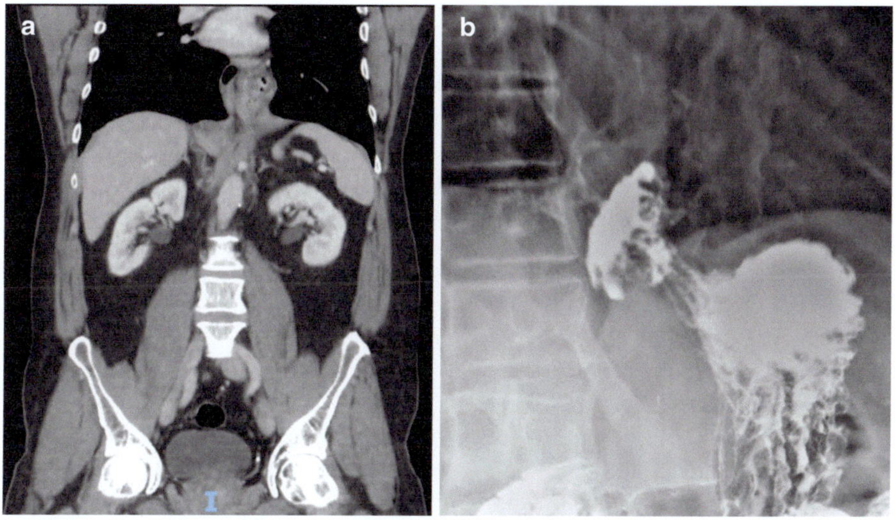

Fig. 3 (**a**) CT scan showing herniated fundoplication. (**b**) Esophagram showing herniated fundoplication

Computed Tomography

A computed tomography (CT) can further help visualizing the esophagus, the stomach, the diaphragm, and the relationship with all the structures around the EGJ, ultimately giving valuable anatomical information. CT is probably the best test to diagnose and evaluate type IV hiatal hernia (Fig. 3).

Esophageal Manometry

Esophageal manometry is useful to assess postoperative integrated relaxation pressures of the lower esophageal sphincter and the quality of the esophageal peristalsis. A high resting LES pressure could suggest the presence of a tight fundoplication. Conversely, a low esophageal sphincter pressure can indicate failure of the fundoplication or recurrence of hiatal hernia. In addition, the manometry can potentially identify primary esophageal motility disorders than were misdiagnosed initially.

Ambulatory pH Monitoring

This study is the gold standard to confirm if the patient has pathologic gastroesophageal reflux or not. In addition, it helps determining whether reflux episodes are associated with patient's complaints (correlation between reflux episodes and main symptoms of the patient) [18].

Management

The treatment of patients with failed ARS largely depends on the mechanism of failure. As previously discussed, a thorough diagnostic work-up can eventually elucidate if there was a poor judgment of the surgeon regarding patient selection (e.g. misdiagnosis of reflux with other digestive disorders). After a complete diagnostic evaluation, patients should be counseled about the different medical, endoscopic and surgical options.

Patients with anatomical failures and persistent/recurrent symptoms will likely require an operation. However, optimizing medical therapy and evaluating response to medication remains a reasonable first approach in most patients. Surgical revision should be reserved for patients with significant symptom burden that is not well controlled with PPI.

Redo ARS is significantly more complex than a primary fundoplication, mostly due to altered anatomy and adhesions. As redo anti-reflux surgery is associated with significantly higher morbidity, it is important to have an extensive and detailed discussion with the patient regarding the risks of the operation (esophageal/gastric perforation, bleeding, vagal nerve injury) [19, 20]. In expert hands, however, laparoscopic revisional fundoplication is a safe procedure with a low rate of complications and satisfactory long-terms results [21].

The most common redo procedure involves removing the previous fundoplication, performing a redo fundoplication, and repairing the recurrent hiatal hernia if present [22].

In the case of a tight fundoplication and an intact wrap below the diaphragm, endoscopic dilation is an option. Esophageal dilation should begin with smaller balloon sizes, such as 10–20 mm, and can be progressively increased over several sessions to reduce the risk of complications. [23, 24]. In cases of refractory dysphagia, a surgical revision may be required.

In cases where a short esophagus contributed to the primary failure of fundoplication, a redo fundoplication with Collis gastroplasty should be performed. The use of mesh in the hiatus during revisional surgery is debated, but it should be considered when poor quality of the muscle of the crura is identified [25]. In severe cases of gastroparesis due to vagal disruption, a pyloroplasty might be necessary. A Roux-en-Y gastric bypass is also an option following failed ARS, especially in patients with obesity [26].

A treatment algorithm for patients with persistent/recurrent symptoms after ARS is proposed by our study group (Fig. 4).

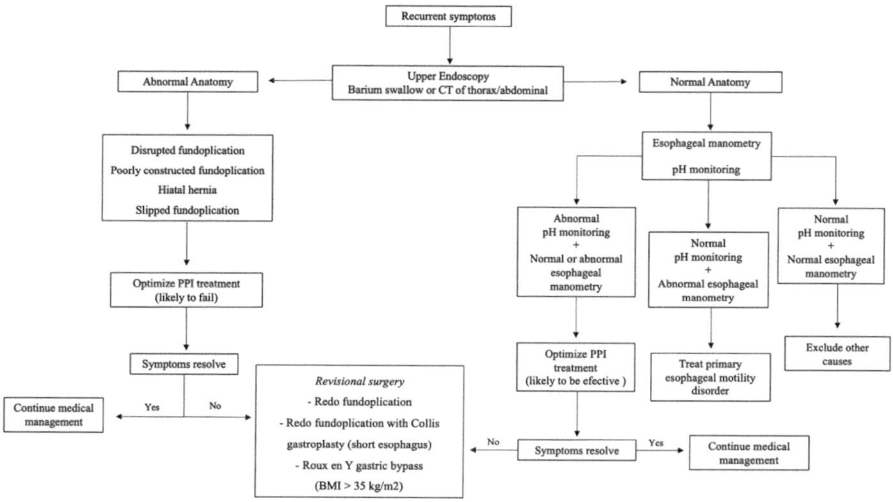

Fig. 4 Management of patients with recurrent symptoms after anti-reflux surgery

Conclusions

Laparoscopic ARS is an effective therapy for GERD with long-term successful outcomes. Some patients, however, will be affected by troublesome symptoms after the operation. A failed antireflux procedure is often related to poor surgeon's judgement, anatomical failures, and/or physiological failures. It is critical to perform a thorough diagnostic work-up to elucidate the mechanism of failure and offer a tailored therapy for each patient.

Conflict of Interest The authors have no conflicts of interest.

References

1. Dallemagne B, Weerts J, Markiewicz S, et al. Clinical results of laparoscopic fundoplication at ten years after surgery. Surg Endosc. 2006;20(1):159–65.
2. Morgenthal CB, Shane MD, Stival A, et al. The durability of laparoscopic Nissen fundoplication: 11-year outcomes. J Gastrointest Surg. 2007;11(6):693–700.
3. Robinson B, Dunst CM, Cassera MA, et al. 20 years later: laparoscopic fundoplication durability. Surg Endosc. 2015;29:2520–4.
4. Li G, Jiang N, Chendaer N, et al. Laparoscopic Nissen versus Toupet fundoplication for short- and long-term treatment of gastroesophageal reflux disease: a meta-analysis and systematic review. Surg Innov. 2023;30(6):745–57.
5. Fisichella PM, Schlottmann F, Patti MG. Evaluation of gastroesopheal reflux disease. Updates Surg. 2018;70(3):309–13.
6. Patti MG, Diener U, Tamburini A, et al. Role of esophageal function tests in diagnosis of gastroesophageal reflux disease. Dig Dis Sci. 2001;46(3):597–602.

7. Pauwels A, Boecxstaens V, Andrews CN, et al. How to select patients for antireflux surgery? The ICARUS guidelines (international consensus regarding preoperative examinations and clinical characteristics assessment to select adult patients for antireflux surgery). Gut. 2019;68(11):1928–41.
8. Campos GM, Peters JH, DeMeester TR, et al. Multivariate analysis of factors predicting outcome after laparoscopic Nissen fundoplication. J Gastrointest Surg. 1999;3(3):292–300.
9. Booth MI, Stratford J, Jones L, Dehn TCB. Randomized clinical trial of laparoscopic total (Nissen) versus posterior partial (Toupet) fundoplication for gastro-oesophageal reflux disease based on preoperative oesophageal manometry. Br J Surg. 2008;95(1):57–63.
10. Horgan S, Pohl D, Bogetti D, Eubanks T, Pellegrini C. Failed antireflux surgery: what have we learned from reoperations? Arch Surg. 1999;134(8):809–17.
11. Peters JH, DeMeester TR, Crookes P, et al. The treatment of gastroesophageal reflux disease with laparoscopic Nissen fundoplication. Ann Surg. 1998:22840–50.
12. Soper NJ, Dunnegan D. Anatomic fundoplication failure after laparoscopic antireflux surgery. Ann Surg. 1999;229(5):669–76. discussion 676–7
13. Awais O, Luketich JD, Schuchert MJ, et al. Reoperative antireflux surgery for failed fundoplication: an analysis of outcomes in 275 patients. Ann Thorac Surg. 2011;92(3):1083–9. discussion 1089–90
14. Tian ZC, Wang B, Shan CX, et al. A meta-analysis of randomized controlled trials to compare long-term outcomes of Nissen and Toupet Fundoplication for gastroesophageal reflux disease. PLoS One. 2015;10(6):e0127627.
15. Lin DC, Chun CL, Triadafilopoulos G. Evaluation and management of patients with symptoms after anti-reflux surgery. Dis Esophagus. 2015;28(1):1–10.
16. Pessaux P, Arnaud JP, Delattre JF, et al. Laparoscopic antireflux surgery: five-year results and beyond in 1340 patients. Arch Surg. 2005;140(10):946–51.
17. van Rijn S, Roebroek YG, Conchillo JM, et al. Effect of Vagus nerve injury on the outcome of antireflux surgery: an extensive literature review. Dig Surg. 2016;33(3):230–9.
18. Yadlapati R, Hungness ES, Pandolfino JE. Complications of antireflux surgery. ACG. 2018;113(8):1137–47.
19. Singhal S, Kirkpatrick DR, Masuda T, et al. Primary and redo antirefux surgery: outcomes and lessons learned. J Gastrointest Surg. 2018;22:177–86.
20. Maret-Ouda J, Wahlin K, El-Serag HB, Lagergren J. Association between laparoscopic antireflux surgery and recurrence of gastroesophageal reflux. JAMA. 2017;318(10):939–46.
21. Siemssen B, Hentschel F, Ibach MJ. Long-term results after laparoscopic revision fundoplication: a retrospective, single-center analysis in 194 patients with recurrent hiatal hernia. Esophagus. 2024;21(3):390–6.
22. Furnée EJ, Draaisma WA, Broeders IA, Gooszen HG. Surgical reintervention after failed antireflux surgery: a systematic review of the literature. J Gastrointest Surg. 2009;13(8):1539–49.
23. Athanasiadis DI, Selzer D, Stefanidis D, et al. Postoperative dysphagia following esophagogastric fundoplication: does the timing to first dilation matter? J Gastrointest Surg. 2021;25(11):2750–6.
24. Salehi N, Cygiel G, Marshall T, et al. Clinical outcomes of endoscopic balloon dilation for dysphagia after anti-gastroesophageal reflux surgery. Surg Endosc. 2024:1–7.
25. Laxague F, Sadava EE, Herbella F, Schlottmann F. When should we use mesh in laparoscopic hiatal hernia repair? A systematic review. Dis Esophagus. 2020; epub ahead of print
26. Castillo-Larios R, Gunturu NS, Cornejo J, et al. Redo fundoplication vs. Roux-en-Y gastric bypass conversion for failed anti-reflux surgery: which is better? Surg Endosc. 2023;37(8):6429–37.

Why Does Fundoplication Fail?

Fernando A. Herbella, Francisco Schlottmann,
and Marco G. Patti

Introduction

Laparoscopic fundoplication is a very successful treatment modality for patients with gastroesophageal reflux disease (GERD) with control of symptoms in about 80–90% of patients [1, 2]. However, about 10–20% of patients experience persistence or recurrence of their symptoms and eventually between 3% and 6% need a second antireflux operation [3, 4].

Most experts would agree that failure of a fundoplication to resolve symptoms is generally due to one of the following causes: (1) wrong indications for the operation; (2) wrong preoperative workup; and (3) failure to execute the proper technical steps.

Indications for Antireflux Surgery

- Heartburn as the main symptom with good response to medical therapy

Contrary to the common belief that patients with poor response to medical therapy are good candidates for surgery, the presence of typical symptoms such as heartburn with good response to medications is a strong predictor of success of fundoplication. For instance, Campos et al. showed that the three factors that were predictive

F. A. Herbella
Department of Surgery, Federal University of São Paulo, São Paulo, São Paulo, Brazil
e-mail: herbella.dcir@epm.br

F. Schlottmann
University of Buenos Aires, Ciudad Autónoma Buenos Aires, Buenos Aires, Argentina

M. G. Patti (✉)
Department of Surgery, University of Virginia Hospital, Charlottesville, VA, USA

F. Schlottmann et al. (eds.), *Esophageal Disorders*,
https://doi.org/10.1007/978-3-032-08179-7_8

of a successful outcome after a fundoplication were the presence of typical symptoms, clinical response to acid suppression therapy, and an abnormal 24-h pH monitoring score [5]. The findings of this study were confirmed by the ICARUS guidelines, an international consensus regarding preoperative examinations and clinical characteristics assessment to select adult patients for antireflux surgery [6]. Specifically, patients with a good response to proton pump inhibitors (PPI) were considered excellent candidates for antireflux surgery and this was the only grade A recommendation among many guidelines [6].

- Regurgitation not responsive to medical therapy

Proton pump inhibitors reduce the acid production of the parietal cells but have no effect on the lower esophageal sphincter (LES) so that regurgitation can still occur despite PPI therapy.

- GERD symptoms and large hiatal hernia

Patients with large hiatal hernias often have GERD symptoms that can persist despite medical therapy. A recent study investigated how the size of a hiatal hernia affects the degree of mucosal injury, the esophageal function, and the reflux profile, [7]. Specifically, the increasing size of the hiatal hernia was associated with more severe esophagitis, lower pressure of the LES, weaker peristalsis, and more acid reflux in both the distal and the proximal esophagus. Consequently, patients with large hiatal hernia (>5 cm) had more frequent episodes of coughing and wheezing suggesting respiratory involvement. As medications are not able to correct the altered anatomy of the gastroesophageal junction, symptomatic patients with large hiatal hernia should be considered for antireflux surgery.

- Poor adherence to medical therapy

Long-term PPI prescribing in general practice is common. However, only a minority of patients request their prescription regularly and this is mostly due to fear of side effects, lack of knowledge about the drugs, and desire to remain in personal control [8].

- Side effects of medical treatment

There is some evidence in the literature that long-term use of PPI might be associated with side effects such as acute interstitial nephritis, chronic kidney disease, hypomagnesaemia, dementia, cardiovascular events and pneumonia [9, 10].

- Barrett's esophagus and antireflux surgery

Based on the existing data, and until a properly conducted multicenter prospective and randomized trial is performed, we do not recommend LARS in patients with BE metaplasia to avoid progression to dysplasia and cancer. As stressed by the guidelines of the American Gastroenterological Association, antireflux surgery should not be considered as an antineoplastic measure in patients with BE [11]. The indications for surgery should be the same as for the treatment of GERD without BE as described before.

Wrong Preoperative Workup

Proper patient selection is critical to achieve excellent results after antireflux surgery. A key element is an accurate preoperative workup that should include a symptomatic evaluation (including the evaluation of the response to PPI therapy), barium swallow, upper endoscopy, esophageal manometry, and ambulatory pH monitoring. A gastric emptying study should be performed in selected patients only. This is an evidence and experience-based consensus recommendation of the Esophageal Diagnostic Advisory Panel composed by expert gastroenterologists and surgeons [12]. Overall, each test has a specific role in the workup and diagnosis of GERD, but no single test alone can provide the entire clinical picture.

- Limitations of symptomatic evaluation

Many physicians believe that that GERD can be diagnosed by clinical history and that additional tests are not necessary. However, many studies have shown that even typical symptoms such as heartburn and regurgitation have low accuracy leading to a wrong diagnosis of GERD in 30–50% of patients [13, 14]. For instance, Patti et al. found that among 822 consecutive patients referred for esophageal function tests because of a clinical diagnosis of GERD (based on symptoms and endoscopic findings—patients with biopsy proven Barrett's esophagus were excluded), abnormal reflux by pH monitoring was present in 70% of patients only [13]. Heartburn and regurgitation were equally frequent in patients with and without an abnormal pH monitoring study. Many patients with a normal esophageal acid exposure had been treated with medication on the assumption that gastroesophageal reflux was the cause of their symptoms, masking other diagnoses such as irritable bowel syndrome gallstone disease, and even coronary artery disease. In addition, some patients who had been referred for antireflux surgery because they did not improve with PPI therapy ("refractory GERD") were found to have achalasia.

Bello et al. analyzed the sensitivity and specificity of symptoms, endoscopy, barium esophagogram and manometry as compared with ambulatory pH monitoring in 138 patients referred for antireflux surgery [15]. Four patients were excluded as they were found to have achalasia. Of the remaining 134 patients, 56 (42%) had normal pH monitoring results and 78 (58%) had a pathologic amount of reflux. When these two groups were compared, the was no difference in the incidence of symptoms, presence of reflux and hiatal hernia on esophagogram, endoscopic findings and esophageal motility. This study clearly indicated that symptoms are unreliable in diagnosing GERD, the presence of reflux or hiatal hernia on esophagogram does not correlate with the findings of pH monitoring, esophagitis on endoscopy has low sensitivity and specificity, and manometry is mostly useful for positioning of the pH probe and to rule out achalasia [15]. Ambulatory pH monitoring should be routinely performed in patients suspected of having GERD to avoid unnecessary antireflux surgery.

Failure to Respect the Proper Technical Elements

The better understanding of the pathogenesis of GERD in recent years has not been accompanied by appreciable advances in the design of antireflux operations. In many cases operations are still performed just as they were described many decades ago. Today it is important to go beyond the eponymous procedures (Nissen, Toupet, Dor, Guarner, Lind) traditionally associated with antireflux operations, and to identify the technical elements that are important to create an effective and durable fundoplication [16].

- Dissection of the esophagus in the posterior mediastinum

This is a key step as it is important to have 3–5 cm of esophagus without any tension below the diaphragm. Figure 1a shows both the gastroesophageal junction and the wrap located above the diaphragm: this finding is due to very limited mediastinal dissection. Figure 1b shows that the wrap is located below the diaphragm while the

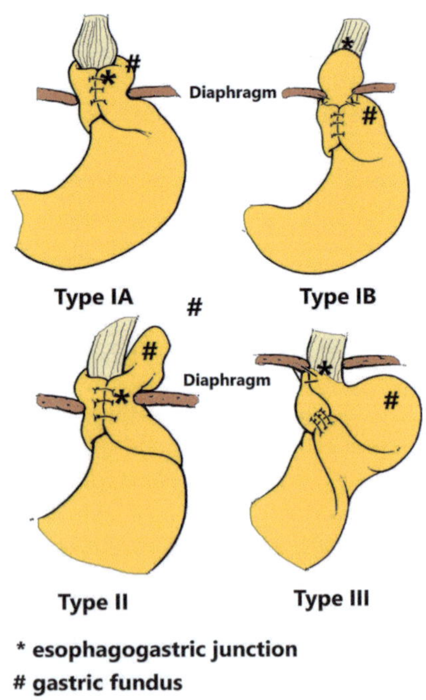

Fig. 1 Anatomic failures of fundoplication as determined during reoperation

gastroesophageal junction is located above: this finding can be due to limited mediastinal dissection, with only 1 or 2 cm of esophagus below the diaphragm, a short esophagus, or inadequate closure of the hiatus.

- Transection of the short gastric vessels

In 2008 Yang et al. published the 10-year results of a randomized trial of division versus non division of the short gastric vessels during laparoscopic Nissen fundoplication [17]. The study showed a similar control of symptoms and incidence of postoperative dysphagia in the two groups. Most surgeons, however, routinely transect the short gastric vessels, as they feel that this is a necessary step that makes it easier to select the proper site in the fundus for the wrap, avoiding tension.

- Approximation of the right and left pillar of the crus

This is an important step (non-absorbable sutures must be used) for two reasons: (1) it avoids herniation of the wrap in the posterior mediastinum [18]; and (2) it re-establishes the synergistic action of the diaphragm with the LES, protecting against sudden increases in intra-abdominal pressure such as during coughing.

- Creation of the wrap over a bougie

We routinely use a 56F to 60F bougie before performing the shoe-shine maneuver. There is some evidence to suggest that both the use and the size of the bougie might help decrease the incidence of postoperative dysphagia [19].

- Shoeshine maneuver

A proper point of the greater curvature of the stomach must be chosen for the wrap. If this is too low, often in the attempt to create "a floppy fundoplication", one of two problems can occur: part of the stomach herniates above the wrap, or the body rather than the fundus of the stomach is used to construct the wrap. A shoeshine maneuver (Fig. 2) can avoid this mistake in most cases. An insightful analysis of the anatomic causes of failure was provided by Horgan et al. from the University of Washington in Seattle [20].

- Fundoplication

In the nineties a tailored approach to antireflux surgery was often followed whereby a total fundoplication (360°) was performed in patients with normal esophageal peristalsis while a partial fundoplication (240°–270°) was chosen if abnormal peristalsis was present [21]. In addition, some single center and retrospective studies suggested that total fundoplication was more effective than partial fundoplication in controlling pathologic reflux and symptoms [22–24].

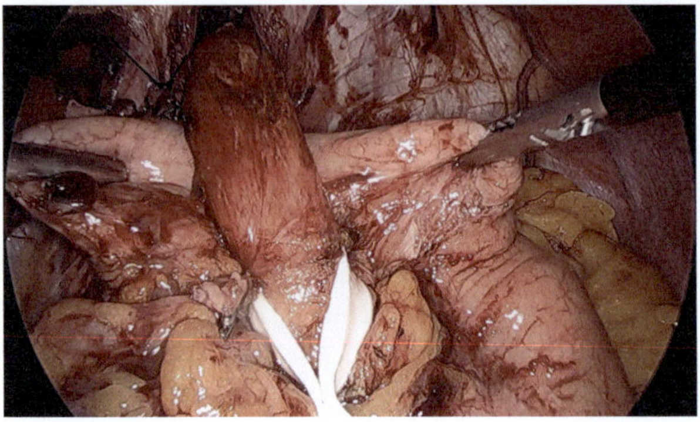

Fig. 2 Shoeshine maneuver

Interestingly, data from Europe and Australia show similar results for both procedures in terms of reflux control and incidence of postoperative dysphagia [25]. Two recent double-blind, randomized clinical trials comparing laparoscopic total versus 270° posterior partial fundoplication confirmed equal control of the reflux and the symptoms, with the suggestion that early postoperative dysphagia might be more common after total fundoplication [26, 27]. Based on these findings, it is up to the individual surgeon to choose the type of laparoscopic fundoplication based on his/her own experience and outcomes.

Evaluation of Patients with Persistent or Recurrent Symptoms

If a patient develops foregut symptoms after a fundoplication, it is assumed that the operation has failed, and acid-reducing medications are often prescribed. A proper workup, including esophageal manometry and ambulatory pH monitoring, is seldom performed early in the management of these patients. Many studies, however, have shown that in patients who are symptomatic after a fundoplication for GERD, a symptom-based diagnosis is not accurate and that a thorough investigation is necessary to determine if the symptoms are due to pathologic reflux, to identify the cause, and tailor treatment.

Lord et al. evaluated with manometry and pH monitoring 86 patients who had foregut symptoms after a Nissen fundoplication [28]. Thirty-seven patients (43%) were taking acid reducing medications. However, only 23% (20 of 86) of all patients and only 24% (9 of 37) of those taking medications had abnormal esophageal acid exposure on the 24-h pH study. Similar results were described by Galvani et al. [29]. Among 124 patients who developed foregut symptoms after laparoscopic fundoplication (average of 17 months postoperatively), only 48 patients (39%) had abnormal esophageal acid exposure. Overall, these studies show that because symptoms have a limited predictive power, objective evidence of reflux disease should be obtained early in the evaluation of these patients after fundoplication to avoid improper and costly medical therapy.

In addition to the symptomatic evaluation (assessing the response to PPI), we routinely perform a barium swallow, endoscopy, manometry and pH monitoring.

The combination of barium swallow and upper endoscopy usually identifies possible anatomic problems such as a herniated wrap or a wrong configuration of the fundoplication.

Esophageal manometry assesses the pressure and relaxation of the LES and the quality of esophageal peristalsis. This is particularly important if the patient experienced severe dysphagia in addition to heartburn preoperatively to rule out achalasia [14].

Ambulatory pH monitoring shows if abnormal reflux is present and assesses the correlation between episodes of reflux and symptoms.

Conclusions

Laparoscopic fundoplication is an excellent treatment modality for patients with GERD. A proper patients' selection is based on solid indications for surgery, a through preoperative workup and an operation that respects the key technical elements.

If the patient experiences persistent or recurrent symptoms, a complete workup is necessary to determine if recurrent reflux is present and identify the cause of the failure.

Conflict of Interest The Author has no conflict of interest to declare.

References

1. Dallemagne B, Weerts J, Markiewicz S, et al. Clinical results of laparoscopic fundoplication at ten years after surgery. Surg Endosc. 2006;20:159–65.
2. Fein M, Bueter M, Thalheimer A, et al. Ten-year outcome of laparoscopic antireflux surgery. J Gastrointest Surg. 2008;12:1893–9.
3. Carlson MA, Frantzides CT. Complications and results of primary minimally invasive antireflux procedures: a review of 10,735 reported cases. J Am Coll Surg. 2001;193:428–39.
4. Catarci M, Gentileschi P, Papi C, et al. Evidence-based appraisal of antireflux fundoplication. Ann Surg. 2004;239:325–37.
5. Campos GM, Peters JH, DeMeester TR, et al. Multivariate analysis of factors predicting outcome after laparoscopic Nissen fundoplication. J Gastrointest Surg. 1999;3:292–300.
6. Pauwels A, Boecxstaens V, Andrews CN, et al. How to select patients for antireflux surgery? The ICARUS guidelines (international consensus regarding preoperative examinations and clinical characteristics assessment to select adults for antireflux surgery). Gut. 2019;68:1928–41.
7. Schlottmann F, Andolfi C, Herbella FA, et al. GERD: presence and size of hiatal hernia influence clinical presentation, esophageal function, reflux profile, and degree of mucosal injury. Am Surg. 2018;84:978–82.
8. Hungin AP, Rubin G, O'Flanagan H. Factor influencing compliance in long-term proton pump inhibitor therapy in general practice. Br J Gen Pract. 1999;49:463–4.

9. Dharmarajan TS. The use and misuse of proton pump inhibitors: an opportunity for deprescribing. J Am Med Dir Assoc. 2021;22:15–22.
10. Rooney MR, Bell EJ, Alonso A, et al. Proton pump inhibitor use, hypomagnesemia and risk of cardiovascular disease: the atherosclerosis risk in communities (ARIC) study. J Clin Gastroenterol. 2021;55:677–83.
11. Shaheen NJ, Falk GW, Iyer PG, et al. Diagnosis and management of Barrett's esophagus: an updated ACG guideline. Am J Gastroenterol. 2022;117:559–87.
12. Jobe BA, Richter JE, Hoppo T, et al. Preoperative diagnostic workup before antireflux surgery: an evidence and experience-based consensus of the Esophageal Diagnostic Advisory Panel. J Am Coll Surg. 2013;217:586–97.
13. Patti MG, Diener U, Tambutini A, Molena D, Way LW. Role of esophageal function tests in the diagnosis of gastroesophageal reflux disease. Dig Dis Sci. 2001;46:597–602.
14. Chan K, Liu G, Miller L, et al. Lack of correlation between a self-administered subjective GERD questionnaire and pathologic GERD diagnosed by 24-h esophageal pH monitoring. J Gastrointest Surg. 2010;14:427–36.
15. Bello B, Zoccali M, Gullo R, et al. Gastroesophageal reflux disease and antireflux surgery-what is the proper work-up? J Gastrointest Surg. 2013;17:14–20.
16. Allaix ME, Herbella FA, Patti MG. Laparoscopic fundoplication for gastroesophageal reflux disease. How I do it. J Gastrointest Surg. 2013;17:822–8.
17. Yang H, Watson DI, Lally CJ, et al. Randomized trial of division of the short gastric vessels during laparoscopic Nissen fundoplication: 10-year outcomes. Ann Surg. 2008;247:38–42.
18. Soper NJ, Dunnegan D. Anatomic fundoplication failure after laparoscopic antireflux surgery. Ann Surg. 1999;229:676–7.
19. Jarral OA, Athanasiou T, Hanna GB, Zacharakis E. Is an intra-oesophageal bougie of use during Nissen fundoplication? Interact Cardiovasc Thorac Surg. 2012;14:828–33.
20. Horgan S, Pohl D, Bogetti D, et al. Failed antireflux surgery. What have we learned from reoperation? Arch Surg. 1999;134:809–17.
21. Patti MG, Arcerito M, Feo C, et al. An analysis of operations for gastroesophageal reflux disease. Identifying the important technical elements. Arch Surg. 1998;133:600–7.
22. Horvath KD, Jobe BA, Dm H, Swanstrom LL. Laparoscopic Toupet fundoplication is an inadequate procedure for patients with severe reflux disease. J Gastrointest Surg. 1999;3:583–91.
23. Oleynikov D, Eubanks TR, Oelschlager BK, Pellegrini CA. Total fundoplication is the operation of choice for patients with gastroesophageal reflux and defective peristalsis. Surg Endosc. 2002;16:909–13.
24. Patti MG, Robinson T, Galvani C, et al. Total fundoplication is superior to partial fundoplication even when esophageal peristalsis is weak. J Am Coll Surg. 2004;198:863–70.
25. Broeders JAJ, Mauritz FA, Ali UA, et al. Systematic review and meta-analysis of laparoscopic Nissen (posterior total) versus Touper (posterior partial) fundoplication fr gastro-oesophageal reflux disease. Br J Surg. 2010;97:1318–30.
26. Hakanson BS, Lundell L, Bylund A, Thorell A. Comparison of laparoscopic 270° posterior partial fundoplication vs total fundoplication for the treatment of gastroesophageal reflux disease. A randomized clinical trial. JAMA Surg. 2019;154:479–86.
27. Analatos A, Hakanson BS, Ansorge C, et al. Clinical outcomes of a laparoscopic total vs a 270° posterior partial fundoplication in chronic gastroesophageal reflux disease. A randomized clinical trial. JAMA Surg. 2022;157:473–80.
28. Lord RVN, Kaminski A, Oberg S, et al. Absence of gastroesophageal reflux disease in a majority of patients taking acid suppressing medications after Nissen fundoplication. J Gastrointest Surg. 2002;6:3–10.
29. Galvani C, Fisichella PM, Gorodner MV, Perretta S, Patti MG. Symptoms are a poor indicator of reflux status after fundoplication for gastroesophageal reflux disease. Arch Surg. 2003;138:514–9.

GERD and Bariatric Surgery

Fernando A. Herbella, Veronica Gorodner, and Marco G. Patti

Gastroesophageal reflux disease (GERD) is a multifactorial disease with a prevalence of 15–20% in the western adult population and between 18% and 28% in the United States [1]. Over the last decades obesity has become an epidemic, and epidemiological data have demonstrated that it is an important risk factor for the development of GERD.

Some pathophysiologic factors are similar in obese and non-obese individuals, while others are more relevant in patients with a high Body Mass Index (BMI).

Figure 1 shows that the stomach is traditionally divided into 3 zones: the antrum with G cells producing gastrin, the body with parietal cells producing acid, and the fundus. It is important to keep in mind the anatomy of the stomach and the physiology of gastric secretion to understand how bariatric operations can be linked to GERD.

F. A. Herbella
Department of Surgery, Federal University of São Paulo, São Paulo, São Paulo, Brazil
e-mail: herbella.dcir@epm.br

V. Gorodner
Bariátrica BA, Buenos Aires, Argentina

M. G. Patti (✉)
Department of Surgery, University of Virginia Hospital, Charlottesville, VA, USA

F. Schlottmann et al. (eds.), *Esophageal Disorders*,
https://doi.org/10.1007/978-3-032-08179-7_9

Fig. 1 Gastric physiology

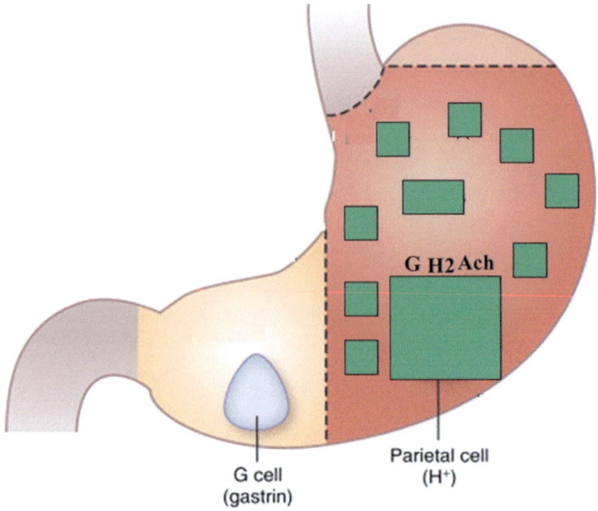

GERD in Obese Patients: Pathophysiology

GERD in the obese may occur due to a defective gastroesophageal barrier or a change in the transdiphragmatic pressure radient (Fig. 2).

- Defective gastroesophageal barrier

While a hypotensive lower esophageal sphincter (LES) is the most common cause of GERD in the general population, it is not always a factor observed in the obese. Some studies found similar LES basal pressures when lean and obese individuals with GERD were compared [2]. Moreover, other studies showed an increased LES basal pressure in the obese, probably linked to compensatory mechanisms due to the increased intra-abdominal pressure [3, 4]. Transient LES relaxations (TLESR), however, seem to be more frequent in the obese, and this might explain GERD in the setting of a normal LES basal pressure. Peristalsis can be impaired with slower esophageal clearance of the refluxate.

Because of deposition of fat at the gastroesophageal junction, common in obese individuals, the angle of His may become obtuse, failing to protect against reflux [5]. Finally, hiatal hernia (HH) is more frequent in the obese [6], and obese women are two and a half times more likely to have HH than non-obese women [7].

- Trans-diaphragmatic pressure gradient

Abdominal pressure is increased in obese individuals due to deposition of abdominal fat, with consequent increase of gastric pressure. For each point of increase in BMI there is a 10% increase in intragastric pressure [8].

Obese patients may also have more negative intrathoracic pressure due to diaphragm elevation secondary to abdominal fat and a consequent decrease in pulmonary expansion. Negative intrathoracic pressure may also be increased by the frequent occurrence of obstructive apnea. Apnea itself may be a cause for GERD due to the increase of TLESR [9].

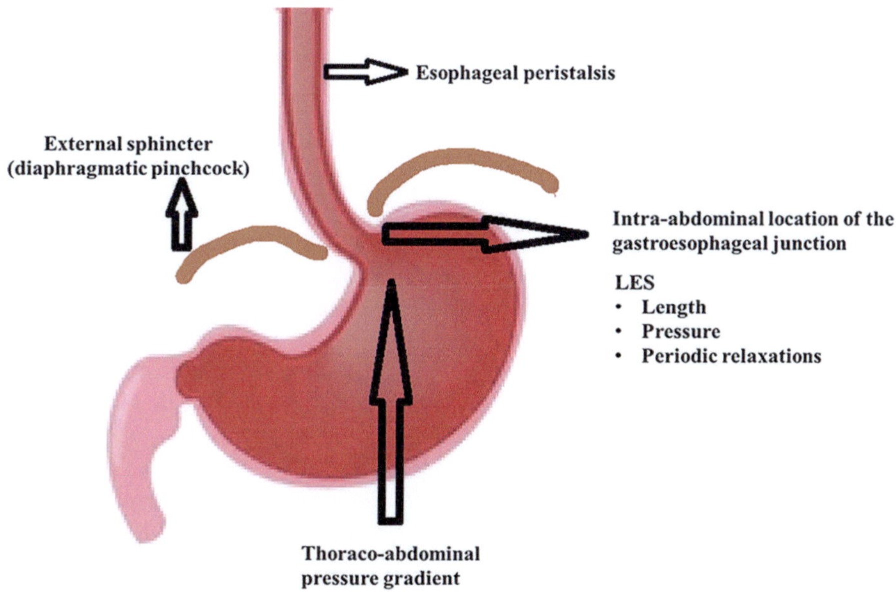

Fig. 2 Pathophysiology of gastroesophageal reflux disease

GERD and Bariatric Operations

The last 2 decades have seen a tremendous increase in the number of bariatric operations performed in the US. While the Roux-en-Y gastric bypass (RYGB) has been for many years the cornerstone of treatment, today the sleeve gastrectomy (SG) is the most common operation. According to data provided by the American Society of Metabolic and Bariatric Surgery (ASMBS), the number of bariatric operations in the US between 2011 and 2022 increased from 150,000/year to 280,000/year [10]: specifically, this study showed a progressive increase of the number of SG over the years, and in 2022 the SG comprised 57.4% of all the procedures, while the RYGB rate was stable at 22.2% of the surgical volume.

Though SG was considered initially the first step of a duodenal switch for super obese patients, today it is used mostly as a solo procedure. The reasons for this shift are multifactorial. Many studies have shown that SG is an effective bariatric operation as it determines weight loss like that of a GB. These results have been recently substantiated by two randomized and multicenter trials performed in Finland and in Switzerland, with large number of patients, and long-term follow-up. Both studies confirmed similar results between RYGB and SG in terms of weight loss [11, 12]. Furthermore, SG is easier and faster to perform than a GB, it does not require anastomoses, it is safer because staple line leaks are infrequent, there is no risk of internal hernias, and it does not preclude the endoscopic exploration of the biliary tract in case of choledocholithiasis, or of the remnant stomach and duodenum for a bleeding ulcer. The two European trials, however, highlighted that while the most common reason for reoperation after RYGB was for treatment of internal hernias, after SG it was for severe reflux refractory to medical treatment, requiring conversion to a RYGB.

Sleeve Gastrectomy

There is today a growing concern that SG may worsen GERD if present preoperatively or might lead to the development of *de novo* GERD [13]. In a large study from Italy with a 5-year follow-up, the mean BMI decreased from 46 to 29 kg/m^2, but postoperatively erosive esophagitis (Los Angeles (LA) grades C and D) developed in 21% of patients, and Barrett's metaplasia in 17% [14]. Interestingly, GERD symptoms were experienced only by 33% of patients with LA grade C esophagitis, and by 57% of patients with LA grade D esophagitis. Others have shown different results. For instance, in a prospective study, Rebecchi et al. showed that the SG improved reflux symptoms in most morbidly obese patients with preoperative GERD, while *de novo* reflux was uncommon [15]. The validity of their conclusions is, however, tempered by the loss of follow-up of about 40% of patients and by the short follow-up of only 2 years. Furthermore, the authors arbitrarily excluded some patients with abnormal pH monitoring as they stated that it was caused by retention of food in the proximal portion of the sleeve. These patients were not considered to have pathological reflux.

GERD after SG is due to one or more of these factors:

(1) loss of the angle of His if the gastric resection is too close to the esophagogastric junction; (2) decrease in the lower esophageal sphincter tone due to resection of sling fibers at the esophagogastric junction, and (3) a decreased gastric compliance and increased intra-gastric pressure secondary to creation of a narrow gastric tube, and to the herniation of part of the gastric sleeve into the posterior mediastinum [16]. Some evidence points out that there is a chance that sleeve gastrectomy may increase the development of *de novo* hiatal hernia [17] secondary to dissection of the angle of His, removal of the fat pad, dissection of the left pillar of the diaphragm, tubular shape of the gastric tube, negative thoracic pressure, rapid weight loss, and fat loss at the level of the crura.

In addition to cases of Barrett's esophagus, recently 3 cases of esophageal adenocarcinoma after SG have been reported [18].

Three male patients had a laparoscopic SG between 2012 and 2015. The preoperative workup had ruled out esophagitis and pathological reflux. All patients were lost to follow-up after 4 months after surgery and were eventually diagnosed with esophageal adenocarcinoma at a mean of 32.5 ± 7.6 months after SG. Patient 1 underwent an esophagectomy with colonic interposition. His final stage was T2N1M1, and died 5 months after surgery. Patient 2 had a subtotal esophagectomy with Roux-en-Y reconstruction and chemotherapy. His final stage was T3N0MX. The third patient was found to have liver metastases (T3N1M1) and did not have surgery. This case report highlights two very important points: (1) patients should have routine endoscopic follow-up after SG regardless of the weight loss and the presence of reflux symptoms; and (2) if a cancer is detected at endoscopy, the patient should be referred to a specialized center for esophagectomy. After a sleeve gastrectomy, only 3 cm to 4 cm of the right gastroepiploic artery are preserved, and the remaining blood supply provided by the right gastric artery may not be sufficient for a gastric pull-up once the left gastric artery is taken down (Fig. 3). In these cases a Roux-en-Y reconstruction or a colonic interposition might be necessary [19].

Roux-en-Y Gastric Bypass

A gastric bypass with Roux-en-Y reconstruction has been traditionally considered an effective bariatric operation in terms of weight loss and resolution of comorbidities. In addition, it often prevents GERD or even correct preexisting GERD because in the small gastric pouch there are very few acid producing parietal cells, and a Roux loop longer than 75–100 cm prevents reflux of bile. For these reasons, it is often used as an antireflux operation in patients who experience recurrent symptoms after fundoplication [20].

There are however many recent studies that have shown that a RYGB is not an infallible antireflux operation as previously thought [21]. Raj et al. studied (by 24-h pH monitoring) 13 patients after SG and 16 patients after RYGB and found

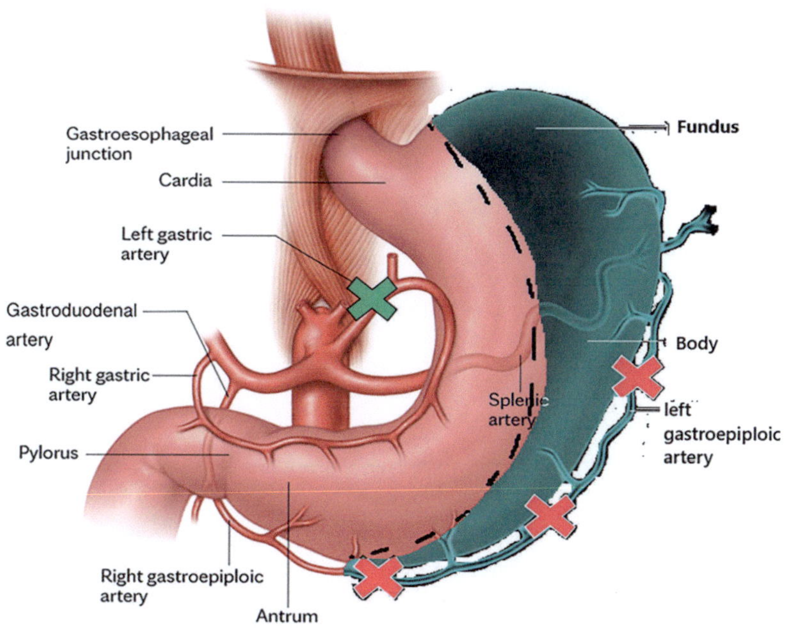

Fig. 3 Gastric blood supply after sleeve gastrectomy and ligation of the left gastric artery to allow lymphadenectomy in cases of cancer after sleeve gastrectomy

pathologic reflux in 66.6% and 12.5% respectively [22]. Navarini et al. found that 1 year after SG and RYGB GERD was more frequent after SG (74% vs 25%) [23]. Similar results were also obtained by a nationwide cohort study in Sweden which assessed the long-term risk of either persisting or recurrent reflux symptoms after RYGB [24]. Among 2454 patients, reflux recurred in 48% of patients within 2 years of the operation. In addition, 68% of patients used antireflux medications during at least one of the first 5 years after the operation.

A very important study was published by Borbely and colleagues from Bern University in Switzerland [25]. This study is germane as it is one of the few studies with a standardized validated questionnaire, upper gastrointestinal studies, endoscopy, manometry and pH monitoring to evaluate patients with symptomatic gastroesophageal reflux after RYGB. Among 47 patients evaluated after a median of 3.8 years after the RYGB, 53% had a hiatal hernia, 10% enlarged pouches, and 5% a gastric/gastric fistula. Endoscopy showed esophagitis and Barrett's esophagus in 51% and 15% of patients respectively. A hypotensive LES was seen in 58% and hypomotility or aperistalsis in 38% of patients undergoing manometry. Finally, pH monitoring showed a pathological amount of reflux in 62% of patients.

GERD after RYGB is probably due to one or more of these factors:

1. The study of Borbely [25] suggested that hiatal hernia, hypotensive LES and severe esophageal motility disorders are key pathophysiologic factors.
2. Size of the gastric pouch. Initially the RYGB was based on a retrocolic/retrogastric Roux loop. Subsequently, the technique evolved to an antecolic/antegastric Roux-loop, technically much simpler. However, because of fear of creating tension of the gastro-jejunal anastomosis, the pouch is often longer than what originally described. Figure 4 clearly illustrates this problem. The stomach was transected at the level of the incisura rather than at the level of the upper border

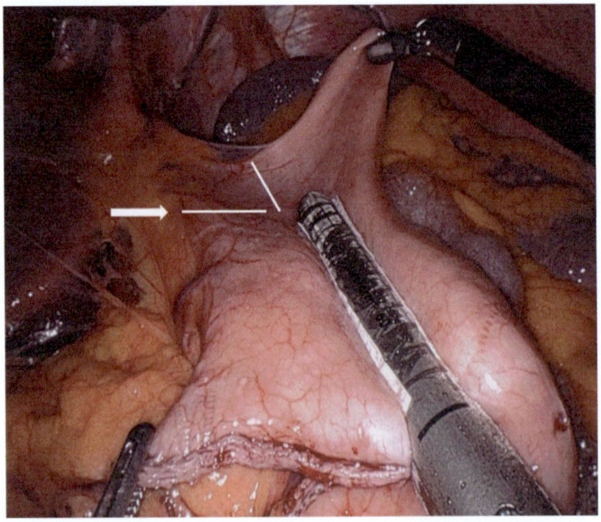

Fig. 4 Very long gastric pouch for Roux-en-Y gastric bypass

of the caudate lobe of the liver, therefore creating a very long pouch, similar in dimension to a sleeve gastrectomy.
3. The length of the Roux loop should be at least 75–100 cm to avoid reflux of bile. A shorter length might allow bile to reflux into the gastric pouch and eventually into the esophagus.

Treatment of GERD After Bariatric Surgery

Treatment depends on the procedure performed and on a thorough work up.

For a sleeve gastrectomy the options include treatment with PPI, magnetic sphincter augmentation, or conversion to a RYGB. If a hiatal hernia is detected, it should be reduced at the time of the operation [26].

For a Roux-en-Y gastric bypass the options include PPI, magnetic sphincter augmentation, or revisional surgery with reduction of hiatal hernia if present, revision of the gastric pouch, and/or length of the Roux loop [27].

Conclusions

- Bariatric surgery is a very effective treatment modality for patients with obesity.
- The success of the operation is based on careful patients' selection including symptom evaluation and endoscopy. In some patients, esophageal manometry and ambulatory pH monitoring are necessary.
- Based on the results of the workup, the appropriate operation must be chosen, usually avoiding SG in patients with preexisting GERD.
- Proper technical steps must be followed.
- Regular follow-up must be established and should be done in every patient after bariatric surgery.

Conflict of Interest The Authors have no conflict of interest to declare.

References

1. El-Serag HB, Sweet S, Winchester CC, Dent J. Update on the epidemiology of gastro-oesophageal reflux disease: a systematic review. Gut. 2014;63:871–80.
2. Valezi AC, Herbella FAM, Schlottmann F, Patti MG. Gastroesophageal reflux disease in obese patients. J Laparoendosc Adv Surg Tech A. 2018;28:949–52.
3. Quiroga E, Cuenca-Abente F, Flum D. Impaired esophageal function in morbidly obese patients with gastroesophageal reflux disease: evaluation with multichannel intraluminal impedance. Surg Endosc. 2006;20:739–43.
4. Herbella FA, Sweet MP, Tedesco P, Nipomnick I, Patti MG. Gastroesophageal reflux disease and obesity. Pathophysiology and implications for treatment. J Gastrointest Surg. 2007;11:286–90.
5. Richter JE, Rubenstein JH. Gstroesophageal reflux disease – presentation and epidemiology of gastroesophageal reflux disease. Gastroenterology. 2018;154:267–76.

6. Valezi AC, Herbella FA, Mali J Jr. Gastroesophageal reflux disease: pathophysiology. In: Fisichella PM, Allaix ME, Morino M, Patti MG, editors. Esophageal diseases. Evaluation and treatment. New York: Springer; 2014. p. 41–51.
7. Suter M, Dorta G, Giusti V, et al. Gastro-esophageal reflux and esophageal motility disorders in morbidly obese patients. Obes Surg. 2004;14:959–66.
8. Mushref MA, Srinivasan S. Effect of high fat-diet and obesity on gastrointestinal motility. Ann Transl Med. 2013;1:14–7.
9. Nadaleto BF, Herbella FAM, Patti MG. Gastroesophageal reflux disease in the obese: pathophysiology and treatment. Surgery. 2016;159:475–86.
10. Clapp B, Ponce J, Corbett J, et al. American Society for Metabolic and Bariatric Surgery 2022 estimate of metabolic and bariatric procedures performed in the United States. Surgery for Obesity Related Diseases. 2024;20:425–31.
11. Peterli R, Wolnerhhanssen BK, Vetter D, et al. Laparoscopic sleeve gastrectomy versus Roux-Y gastric bypass for morbid obesity. Three-year outcome of the prospective randomized Swiss multicenter bypass or sleeve study. Ann Surg. 2017;265:466–73.
12. Salminen P, Helmio M, Ovaska J, et al. Effect of laparoscopic sleeve gastrectomy vs laparoscopic Roux-en-Y gastric bypass on weight loss at 5 years among patients with morbid obesity: the SLEEVEPASS randomized clinical trial. JAMA. 2018;319:241–54.
13. Mandeville Y, Looveren R, Vancoillie PJ, et al. Moderating the enthusiasm of sleeve gastrectomy: up to fifty percent of reflux symptoms after ten years in a consecutive series of one hundred laparoscopic sleeve gastrectomy. Obes Surg. 2017;27:1797–803.
14. Genco A, Soricelli E, Casella G, et al. Gastroesophageal reflux disease and Barrett's esophagus after laparoscopic sleeve gastrectomy: a possible, underestimated long-term complication. Surg Obes Relat Dis. 2017;13:568–74.
15. Rebecchi F, Allaix ME, Giaccone C, et al. Gastroesophageal reflux disease and laparoscopic sleeve gastrectomy. A physiopathologic evaluation. Ann Surg. 2014;260:909–15.
16. da Silva JD, Santa-Cruz F, Cavalcanti JMS, et al. Incidence of abnormalities of the gastric tube following sleeve gastrectomy and its role on esophagitis progression. Obes Surg. 2023;33:263–7.
17. Saba J, Bravo M, Rivas E, Fernández R, et al. Incidence of de novo hiatal hernia after laparoscopic sleeve gastrectomy. Obes Surg. 2020;30:3730–4.
18. Genco A, Castagneto-Gissey L, Lorenzo M, et al. Esophageal. Surg Obes Relat Dis. 2021;17:848–59.
19. Nobel T, Sewell M, Boerner T, et al. Treatment of esophageal adenocarcinoma in patients with history of bariatric surgery. J Gastrointest Surg. 2024;28:337–42.
20. Castillo-Larios R, Gunturu NS, Cornejo J, et al. Redo fundoplication vs. Roux-en-Y gastric bypass conversion for failed anti-reflux surgery: which is better? Surg Endosc. 2023;37:6429–37.
21. Schlottmann F, Masrur MA, Herbella FAM, Patti MG. Roux-en-Y gastric bypass and gastroesophageal reflux disease: an infallible anti-reflux operation? Obes Surg. 2022;32:2481–3.
22. Raj PP, Bhattacharya S, Misra S, et al. Gastroesophageal reflux-related physiologic changes after sleeve gastrectomy and Roux-en-Y gastric bypass: a prospective comparative study. Surg Obes Relat Dis. 2019;15:1261–9.
23. Navarini D, Madalosso CAS, Tognon AP, et al. Predictive factors of gastroesophageal reflux disease in bariatric surgery: a controlled trial comparing sleeve gastrectomy with gastric bypass. Obes Surg. 2020;30:1360–7.
24. Holberg D, Santoni G, Xie S, Lagergren J. Gastric bypass surgery in the treatment of gastrooesophageal reflux symptoms. J Aliment Pharmacol Ther. 2019;50:159-166.
25. Borbely Y, Kroll D, Nett PC, et al. Radiologic, endoscopic, and functional patterns in patients with symptomatic gastroesophageal reflux disease after Roux-en-Y gastric bypass. Surg Obes Relat Dis. 2018;14:764–8.
26. Liu G, Wang P, Ran S, Xue X, Meng H. Surgical treatment strategies for gastroesophageal reflux after laparoscopic sleeve gastrectomy. Front Endocrinol. 2024;15:1–8.
27. Peristeri DV, Rowdhwal SS. Persistent gastroesophageal reflux disease after RYGB: what shall we do next? Surg Innov. 2025;32:62–71.

Achalasia: Diagnostic Evaluation

Rafael C. Katayama, Fernando A. M. Herbella, Francisco Schlottmann, and Marco G. Patti

Introduction

Achalasia is a primary esophageal motility disorder defined by lack of peristalsis and relaxation of the lower esophageal sphincter. It is generally deemed a rare disease [1], although most professionals dealing with the digestive system have seen at least one case. Probably using this assumption of rarity as an excuse, achalasia is frequently misdiagnosed. Almost half of the patients in a series of achalasia were on antacid medication due to an erroneous diagnosis of gastroesophageal reflux disease (GERD) [2] and, more concerning, 4% of patients with achalasia underwent antireflux surgery wrongly diagnosed as GERD [3]. On the other hand, tumors at the esophagogastric junction (EGJ) may lead to pseudoachalasia [3] and lead to erroneous treatment [4]. Not only GERD is included as possible inaccurate diagnosis for achalasia, cases of anorexia [5], presbyesophagus [6], eosinophilic esophagitis and other ENT-, psychiatric, neurologic, cardiologic or thyroid diseases [7] false diagnosis have been reported. A 5-year delay in diagnosing may occur [7]. Thus, this disease diagnosis demands suspicion and a complete workup.

A complete work-up not only gives the correct diagnosis of the disease but also may classify the disease, provide prognosis and guide tailored therapy.

R. C. Katayama · F. A. M. Herbella (✉)
Department of Surgery, Federal University of São Paulo, São Paulo, Brazil
e-mail: herbella.dcir@epm.br

F. Schlottmann
University of Buenos Aires, Ciudad Autónoma Buenos Aires, Buenos Aires, Argentina

M. G. Patti
Department of Surgery, University of Virginia Hospital, Charlottesville, VA, USA

F. Schlottmann et al. (eds.), *Esophageal Disorders*,
https://doi.org/10.1007/978-3-032-08179-7_10

Table 1 Eckardt score to grade achalasia symptoms based on the presence and frequency of common complaints

Score	Dysphagia	Regurgitation	Chest pain	Weight loss (kg)
0	None	None	None	None
1	Occasional	Occasional	Occasional	<5
2	Daily	Daily	Daily	5–10
3	Each meal	Each meal	Each meal	>10

Based on Eckardt et al. [8]

Symptoms

Symptoms of achalasia are associated with the lack of peristalsis and outflow obstruction at the EGJ, leading to dysphagia and regurgitation. Obstruction can result in weight loss due to inadequate nutrition, halitosis due to food retained in the esophagus, and heartburn due to food fermentation and acid production in the esophagus. Uncoordinated contractions may cause chest pain, while aspiration of esophageal contents can lead to coughing. **Dysphagia, regurgitation, and weight loss** are commonly observed in patients with achalasia and constitutes the classical triad of symptoms.

The Eckardt score [8] is a widely used and validate [9, 10] grading system for assessing these symptoms where the presence and frequency of dysphagia, regurgitation, chest pain and weight loss are graded on a score of 0 to 3, with a maximum score of 12. Symptoms are frequently considered relevant with a final score > 3 (Table 1).

Upper Digestive Endoscopy

Upper digestive endoscopy is necessary when achalasia is suspected or diagnosed [11]. However, the diagnosis of the disease is not made by endoscopy. The test appears normal in approximately half of the cases, while only indirect signs are observed in the remaining cases, such as food residue in the esophagus despite adequate fasting time, areas of leukoplasia, and a "puckering" at the gastroesophageal junction (Fig. 1). The endoscopist may notice esophageal dilatation in cases with significant dilatation.

The primary reason for performing an endoscopy is to exclude other associated diseases leading to a similar scenario but called pseudoachalasia or esophageal cancer, since symptoms may be similar, and achalasia is a premalignant condition increasing the risk of squamous cell carcinoma [12].

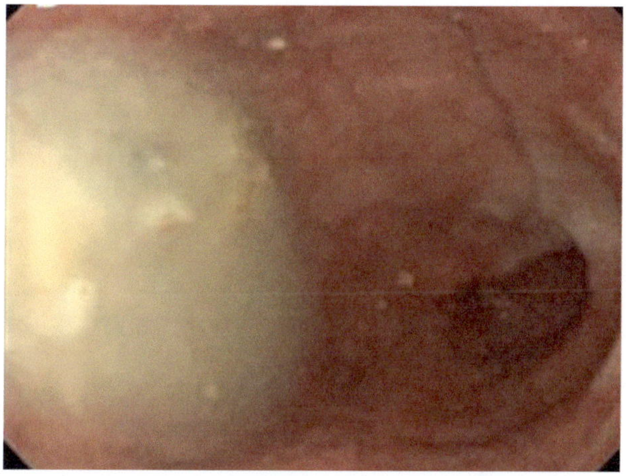

Fig. 1 Endoscopic findings in achalasia (food residue in the esophagus despite adequate fasting time)

Barium Swallow (Esophagram)

A barium esophagogram is a straightforward test used to diagnose and grade esophageal disease. We consider it essential even if the disease has been diagnosed by other methods since the esophagogram also can serve as a baseline measurement of the esophageal diameter for comparison after therapy, especially in cases of treatment failure, identifying if a progression in diameter occurred. Apart from the diagnosis, the degree of esophageal dilatation helps in grading the disease and identifying end-stage disease [13].

The typical findings are a tapering of the distal esophagus (bird's beak sign) and esophageal dilatation (Fig. 2). Associate findings are the presence of food residues, more than 1 air/fluid/fluid levels, tertiary contractions and contrast retention and delay to pass to the stomach.

A massively dilated esophagus (Fig. 3) with bird's beak sign typically has no significant differential diagnosis. Small dilatation without a bird's beak sign can be seen in connective tissue diseases with aperistalsis or end-stage GERD also with aperistalsis or weak peristalsis. Less pronounced esophageal dilatation with tapering may result from tumoral obstruction and pseudoachalasia.

The timed barium swallow test enhances the conventional barium esophagogram by measuring the contrast column after a predetermined volume ingestion and time to assess esophageal emptying. It can be useful in ambiguous cases, but it is more frequently used following treatment [14].

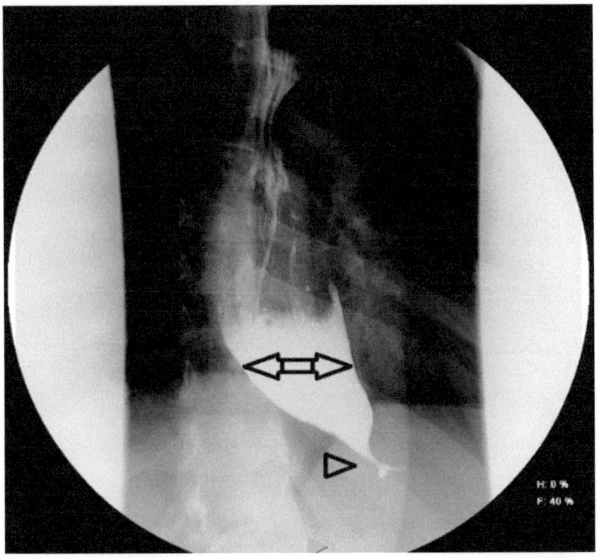

Fig. 2 Barium swallow esophagram findings in achalasia: esophageal dilatation (double arrow) and bird's beak sign (arrowhead)

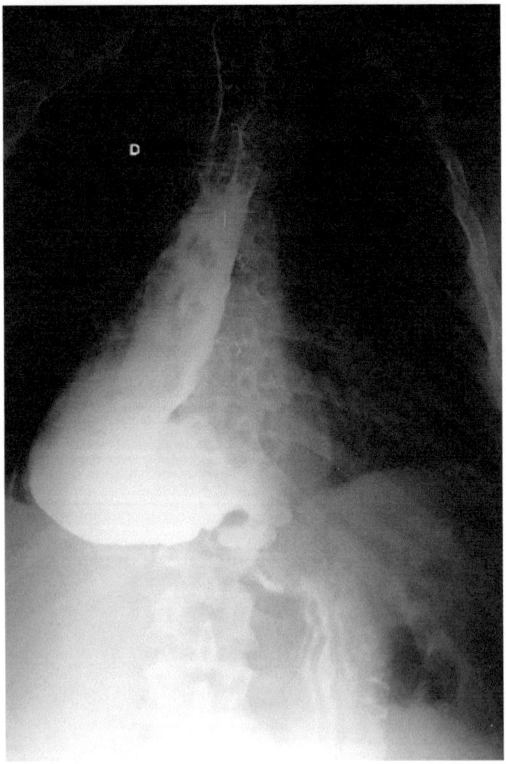

Fig. 3 Massive dilated megaesophagus in achalasia with sigmoid shape of the organ

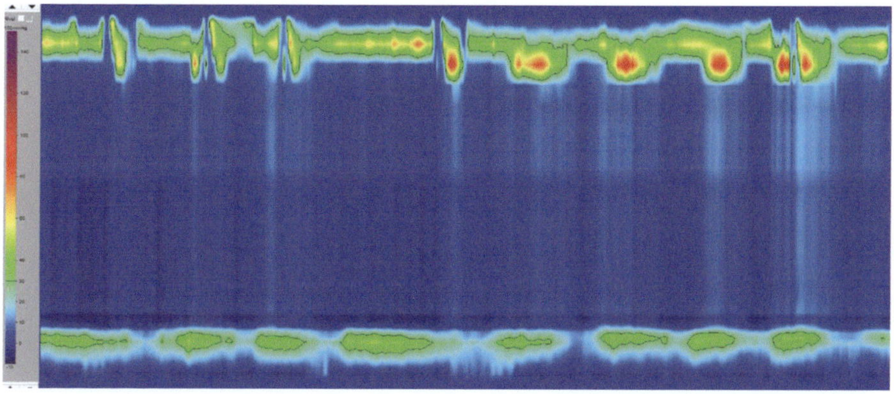

Fig. 4 Achalasia Chicago Type I. Non-relaxing lower esophageal sphincter and failed contractions and no esophageal pressurization

Esophageal Manometry

Esophageal manometry is considered the gold standard test for the diagnosis of achalasia. Even though a barium swallow esophagram may unequivocally give the diagnosis, esophageal manometry can be assertive in dubious cases and also classify the disease according to the Chicago Classification, the current classification of esophageal motility disorders and test performance [15] that has prognostic interest and may guide therapy according to some. The own definition of achalasia is given by manometry: lack of peristalsis and lower esophageal sphincter failure to relax.

Achalasia is defined by a failure of the lower esophageal sphincter (LES) to relax completely and the presence of 100% simultaneous waves, as seen in conventional manometry. Although high-resolution manometry uses a more complex measure called integrated relaxation pressure (IRP), the definition remains unchanged [16].

The Chicago Classification identifies three types of achalasia based on esophageal pressurization during swallows [17] (Figs. 4, 5, and 6). This classification is popular because it links to prognosis and can guide therapy. However, numerous variants were described but without clear treatment guidelines, and insufficient studies resulting in low level of recommendations [18]. These variants denote an inconclusive diagnosis and demand further investigation with other tests. They are: (1) absent contractility with no appreciable peristalsis in the setting of IRP values at the upper limit of normal in both positions, with or without panesophageal pressurization in 20% or more swallows; (2) appreciable peristalsis with changing position in the setting of a type I or II achalasia pattern in the primary position; and (3) abnormal IRP with evidence of spasm and evidence of peristalsis. Again, the evidence provided is low [19].

The complexity of aperistalsis variants results in an interobserver agreement for diagnosing achalasia between 75–84%, even among experienced interpreters [20]. It is too early to determine if artificial intelligence will improve these numbers [21].

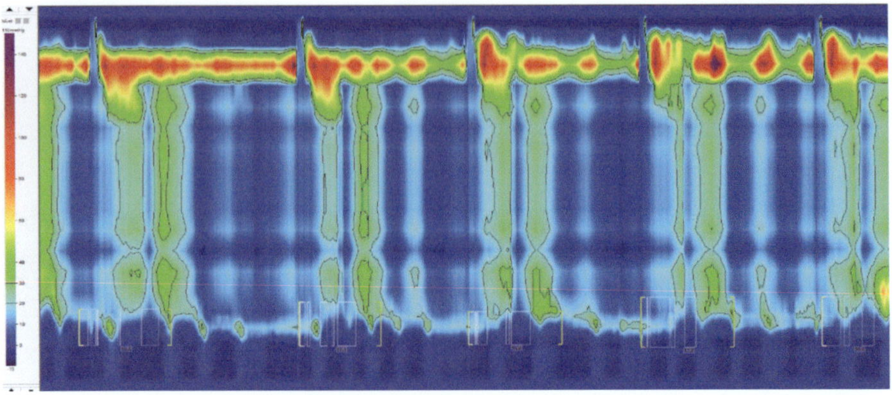

Fig. 5 Achalasia Chicago Type II. Non-relaxing lower esophageal sphincter and failed contractions but panesophageal pressurization in at least 20% of swallows

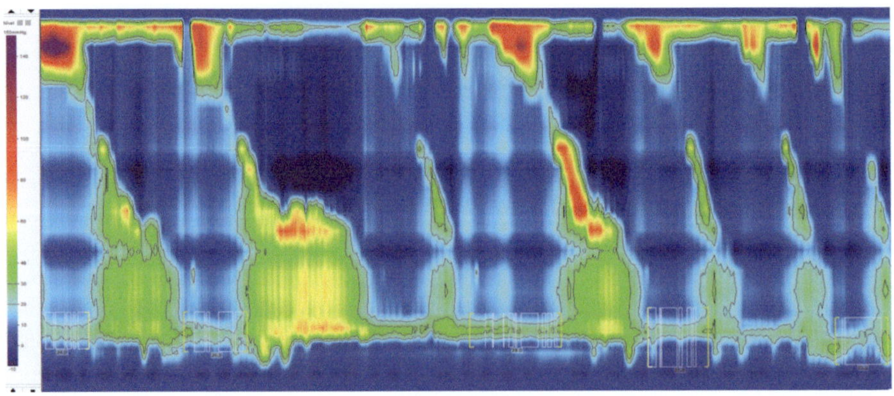

Fig. 6 Achalasia Chicago Type II. Non-relaxing lower esophageal sphincter and failed contractions but premature contractions in at least 20% of swallows

pH Monitoring

GERD is paradoxical in treatment-naive cases because the lack of LES relaxation prevents flux and reflux. However, pseudoreflux may occur due to intraluminal food fermentation and intrinsic acid production leading to false-positive tests. It is easily recognized by the presence of very long nocturnal episodes of esophageal acidification and almost absent reflux in the upright position (Fig. 7) [12].

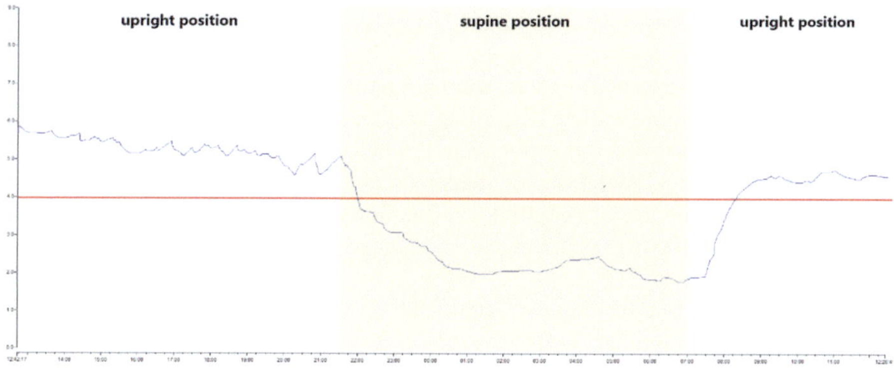

Fig. 7 Pseudoreflux in a patient with achalasia seen as very long nocturnal episodes of esophageal acidification and almost absent reflux in the upright position

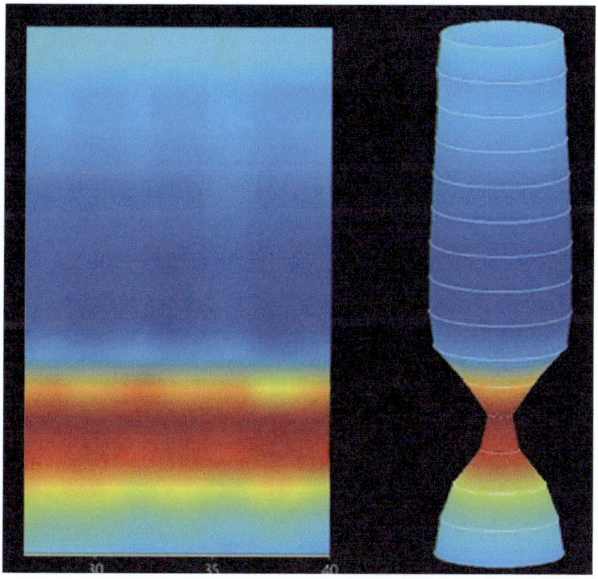

Fig. 8 Endolumenal functional lumen imaging probe (EndoFLIP) measurement of the esophagogastric junction compliance

Endolumenal Functional Lumen Imaging Probe

The endolumenal functional lumen imaging probe (EndoFLIP) measures EGJ compliance (Fig. 8). According to the Chicago Classification, it is a supportive test in cases of inconclusive diagnosis [15]. EndoFLIP may identify abnormal EGJ distensibility in patients who exhibit typical achalasia symptoms but lack the classic manometric features of achalasia [22].

Conclusion

Upper endoscopy is essential to rule out malignancy related to achalasia, a premalignant disease. Barium swallow helps diagnose and confirm achalasia and provides a baseline comparison for the esophageal diameter if treatment fails. Esophageal manometry is the gold standard for diagnosis and aids in prognosis and therapy selection. The routine use of endolumenal functional lumen imaging probe remains unclear.

Conflict of Interest The authors have no conflict of interest.

References

1. Zaninotto G, Bennett C, Boeckxstaens G, et al. The 2018 ISDE achalasia guidelines. Dis Esophagus. 2018;31(9) https://doi.org/10.1093/dote/doy071.
2. Fisichella PM, Raz D, Palazzo F, Niponmick I, Patti MG. Clinical, radiological, and manometric profile in 145 patients with untreated achalasia. World J Surg. 2008;32(9):1974–9. https://doi.org/10.1007/s00268-008-9656-z.
3. Zanini LYK, Herbella FAM, Velanovich V, Patti MG. Modern insights into the pathophysiology and treatment of pseudoachalasia. Langenbeck's Arch Surg. 2024;409(1):65. https://doi.org/10.1007/s00423-024-03259-2.
4. Yu WQ, Gao HJ, Zhai LX, Wei YC. Abnormal performance of peroral endoscopic myotomy (POEM): a case misdiagnosed as achalasia of cardia. J Cardiothorac Surg. 2024;19(1):214. https://doi.org/10.1186/s13019-024-02688-w.
5. Gravier V, Naja W, Blaise M, Cremniter D. Achalasia and megaesophagus misdiagnosed as anorexia nervosa. Eur Psychiatry. 1998;13(6):315–6. https://doi.org/10.1016/S0924-9338(98)80050-3.
6. Rosenzweig S, Traube M. The diagnosis and misdiagnosis of achalasia. A study of 25 consecutive patients. J Clin Gastroenterol. 1989;11(2):147–53. https://doi.org/10.1097/00004836-198904000-00007.
7. Müller M, Förschler S, Wehrmann T, Marini F, Gockel I, Eckardt AJ. Atypical presentations and pitfalls of achalasia. Dis Esophagus. 2023;36(10):doad029. https://doi.org/10.1093/dote/doad029.
8. Eckardt VF, Aignherr C, Bernhard G. Predictors of outcome in patients with achalasia treated by pneumatic dilation. Gastroenterology. 1992;103:1732–8. https://doi.org/10.1016/0016-5085(92)91428-7.
9. Taft TH, Carlson DA, Triggs J, Craft J, Starkey K, Yadlapati R, Gregory D, Pandolfino JE. Evaluating the reliability and construct validity of the Eckardt symptom score as a measure of achalasia severity. Neurogastroenterol Motil. 2018;30(6):e13287. https://doi.org/10.1111/nmo.13287.
10. Patti MG, Herbella FA. The evolution of the treatment of esophageal achalasia. Chronicle of a 35-year journey. Cir Esp (Engl Ed). 2024;102(6):340–6. https://doi.org/10.1016/j.cireng.2024.04.001.
11. Laurino-Neto RM, Herbella F, Schlottmann F, Patti M. Evaluation of esophageal achalasia: from symptoms to the Chicago classification. Arq Bras Cir Dig. 2018;31(2):e1376. https://doi.org/10.1590/0102-672020180001e1376.
12. Schlottmann F, Herbella F, Allaix ME, Patti MG. Modern management of esophageal achalasia: from pathophysiology to treatment. Curr Probl Surg. 2018;55(1):10–37. https://doi.org/10.1067/j.cpsurg.2018.01.001.

13. Schlottmann F, Neto RML, Herbella FAM, Patti MG. Esophageal Achalasia: pathophysiology, clinical presentation, and diagnostic evaluation. Am Surg. 2018;84(4):467–72.
14. Sanagapalli S, Plumb A, Lord RV, Sweis R. How to effectively use and interpret the barium swallow: current role in esophageal dysphagia. Neurogastroenterol Motil. 2023;35(10):e14605. https://doi.org/10.1111/nmo.14605.
15. Yadlapati R, Kahrilas PJ, Fox MR, Bredenoord AJ, Prakash Gyawali C, Roman S, et al. Esophageal motility disorders on high-resolution manometry: Chicago classification version 4.0©. Neurogastroenterol Motil. 2021;33(1):e14058. https://doi.org/10.1111/nmo.14058.
16. Herbella FA, Patti MG. Can high resolution manometry parameters for achalasia be obtained by conventional manometry? World J Gastrointest Pathophysiol. 2015;6(3):58–61. https://doi.org/10.4291/wjgp.v6.i3.58.
17. Schlottmann F, Herbella FA, Patti MG. Understanding the Chicago classification: from tracings to patients. J Neurogastroenterol Motil. 2017;23(4):487–94. https://doi.org/10.5056/jnm17026.
18. Khan A, Yadlapati R, Gonlachanvit S, Katzka DA, Park MI, Vaezi M, Vela M, Pandolfino J. Chicago classification update (version 4.0): technical review on diagnostic criteria for achalasia. Neurogastroenterol Motil. 2021;33(7):e14182. https://doi.org/10.1111/nmo.14182.
19. Herbella FAM, Patti MG, Filho RM, et al. How changes in treatment guidelines affect the standard of care: ethical opinions using the Chicago 4.0 classification for Esophageal motility disorders as example. Foregut. 2022;2(2):111–5. https://doi.org/10.1177/26345161221081038.
20. Nayar DS, Khandwala F, Achkar E, Shay SS, Richter JE, Falk GW, Soffer EE, Vaezi MF. Esophageal manometry: assessment of interpreter consistency. Clin Gastroenterol Hepatol. 2005;3(3):218–24. https://doi.org/10.1016/s1542-3565(04)00617-2.
21. Fass O, Rogers BD, Gyawali CP. Artificial Intelligence tools for improving Manometric diagnosis of Esophageal Dysmotility. Curr Gastroenterol Rep. 2024;26(4):115–23. https://doi.org/10.1007/s11894-024-00921-z.
22. Savarino E, di Pietro M, Bredenoord AJ, Carlson DA, Clarke JO, Khan A, Vela MF, Yadlapati R, Pohl D, Pandolfino JE, Roman S, Gyawali CP. Use of the functional lumen imaging probe in clinical Esophagology. Am J Gastroenterol. 2020;115(11):1786–96. https://doi.org/10.14309/ajg.0000000000000773.

Treatment Modalities for Achalasia

Fernando A. Herbella, Francisco Schlottmann, and Marco G. Patti

The last 3 decades have seen significant progress in the diagnosis and treatment of esophageal achalasia. Conventional manometry has been replaced by high resolution manometry which has determined a more precise classification of achalasia in three subtypes, with important treatment implications. Therapy, though still palliative, has evolved tremendously. While pneumatic dilatation was for a long time the main choice of treatment, this approach slowly changed in the nineties when minimally invasive surgery was adopted—initially thoracoscopically and then laparoscopically. And in 2010 the first report of a new endoscopic technique—per oral endoscopic myotomy (POEM)—was published, revamping the interest in the endoscopic treatment of achalasia [1].

In this chapter we will review the diagnostic evaluation of patients suspected of having achalasia, and we will discuss the available treatment modalities, stressing the benefits and risks of each of them. Finally, we will provide a treatment algorithm based on literature and our own experience.

Achalasia: Evaluation

Dysphagia, regurgitation of undigested food, chest pain and weight loss are the most common symptoms in patients with achalasia [2]. Today the *Eckardt score* is the most frequently used grading system for the evaluation of symptoms of achalasia and for assessing the efficacy of treatment. It attributes points (0–3

F. A. Herbella
Department of Surgery, Federal University of São Paulo, São Paulo, São Paulo, Brazil

F. Schlottmann
University of Buenos Aires, Ciudad Autónoma Buenos Aires, Buenos Aires, Argentina

M. G. Patti (✉)
Department of Surgery, University of Virginia Hospital, Charlottesville, VA, USA

F. Schlottmann et al. (eds.), *Esophageal Disorders*,
https://doi.org/10.1007/978-3-032-08179-7_11

points) to 4 symptoms of the disease (dysphagia, regurgitation, chest pain, and weight loss), ranging from 0 to 12. Patients can also have aspiration of esophageal contents with complications such as wheezing, cough, hoarseness, and pneumonia [3].

Esophagogastroduodenoscopy (EGD) is always performed to exclude other causes of dysphagia such as peptic stricture or a tumor. Typical findings are esophageal dilatation and presence of retained food. Esophageal mucosa can be normal or show signs of esophagitis, usually secondary to food stasis or candida infection. In about 30–40% of patients, the EGD is normal.

The barium swallow often shows the characteristic 'bird beak' sign (narrowing at the level of the gastroesophageal junction), delayed passage of the contrast from the esophagus into the stomach, an air-fluid level, and tertiary contractions of the esophagus. The barium swallow, however, fails to show abnormalities in about 30% of patients, particularly in the early stage of the disease. It is also very useful as it shows the diameter and the axis of the esophagus or associated pathology such as an epiphrenic diverticulum.

Traditionally the diagnosis was established by esophageal manometry performed with water perfused catheters. Achalasia was defined by partial or absent LES relaxation and absent esophageal peristalsis. The lower esophageal sphincter (LES) was hypertensive (resting pressure >45 mmHg) in about 50% of patients [2].

Today the gold standard for the diagnosis of achalasia is the high-resolution esophageal manometry (HRM). It enables the measurement of the pressure, length and relaxation of the lower sphincter, and quality of esophageal peristalsis. To confirm the diagnosis of achalasia, it is necessary to document lack of normal esophageal peristalsis and partial or absent LES relaxation. The Chicago classification introduced by Kahrilas and his colleagues in 2008 and today in version 4.0, distinguishes three types of achalasia [4]:

Type I: aperistalsis and absence of esophageal pressurization.
Type II: aperistalsis and pan-esophageal pressurization in at least 20% of swallows.
Type III: premature spastic contractions (distal latency <4.5 s) in at least 20% of swallows.

The Chicago classification helps choose the proper treatment depending on the type of achalasia (pneumatic dilatation, laparoscopic Heller myotomy, or peroral endoscopic myotomy), and has also important prognostic implications (better outcome of treatment for type II).

Ambulatory pH monitoring studies are rarely performed. This test is recommended in selected patients who experience heartburn to distinguish between gastroesophageal reflux disease (GERD) and achalasia. In addition, a pH monitoring study should also be performed whenever possible after treatment, as patients can develop abnormal reflux which is often asymptomatic. This is particularly important for young patients in whom the untreated reflux might cause over the years esophagitis, strictures, Barrett's esophagus and even cancer.

Treatment

Today 3 excellent treatments are available—pneumatic dilatation, laparsocopic Heller myotomy with partial fundoplication, and POEM.

Pneumatic Dilatation

Pneumatic dilatation was the primary treatment modality for many decades, relegating surgery for patients with recurrent symptoms and for addressing complications such as perforation. The advent of minimally invasive surgery changed this approach, particularly in young male patients in whom pneumatic dilatation seemed to be less effective.

A European prospective and randomized trial comparing pneumatic dilatation (starting with a 30 mm balloon and reserving 35 and 40-mm balloons for persistent or recurrent dysphagia) and LHM with a Dor fundoplication was published in 2011. The primary outcome was therapeutic success (a drop in the Eckardt score to ≤3) at the yearly follow-up assessment. After 2 years, the therapeutic success of pneumatic dilatation (86%) or LHM (90%) was similar [5]. At 5-year follow-up there was still no significant difference between the two treatments—84% LHM and 82% pneumatic dilatation—but 25% of pneumatic dilatation patients required addition dilatations [6]. Even though these results suggested that these treatment modalities are equivalent, some limitations of this trial need to be stressed. First, the protocol was revised during the study period, changing the initial pneumatic dilatation technique using a 35 mm balloon to a 30 mm balloon after the observation of a 31% perforation rate with the 35 mm balloon. Second, expert gastroenterologists performed the pneumatic dilatation while the skills and experience of the surgeons involved in the study were questionable as they were required to have performed just 5 myotomies to participate. In addition, the mucosal perforation rate during LHM was 11%, very high in general and particularly in the absence of previous treatment. Subgroup analysis showed that patients younger than 40 years had better results with LHM.

Finally, the applicability of the findings of this study to practice in the USA and abroad is questionable. Because of the extensive use of LHM during the last 15 years and POEM in the last 10 years, the training and expertise for pneumatic dilation has faded away considerably. Consequently, it seems that today the pendulum has swung towards either LHM or POEM as initial treatment for achalasia; in our practice we reserve pneumatic dilatation for the treatment of recurrent dysphagia after either LHM or POEM.

Laparoscopic Heller Myotomy with Partial Fundoplication

The last 3 decades have witnessed major changes in the surgical treatment of achalasia, moving from an open operation performed through a laparotomy or thoracotomy to a minimally invasive approach.

The first minimally invasive operation in the United States was performed in January of 1991 by surgeons at the University of California San Francisco through a left thoracoscopic approach (thoracoscopic Heller myotomy—THM) [7]. The myotomy extended for a total of 7–8 cm, but only for 0.5 cm onto the gastric wall, without a fundoplication. The results of the first 17 patients operated with this technique indicated that while the operation relieved symptoms in 90% of patients, it was associated with postoperative pathological reflux, as tested by pH monitoring, in 60% of them. Subsequent studies showed that a laparoscopic approach, with the addition of fundoplication, provided similar relief of symptoms while limiting the incidence of postoperative pathological reflux. For instance, Patti et al. compared the outcomes of 30 patients who had a thoracoscopic myotomy (THM) to that of 30 patients who had a LHM with Dor fundoplication. Excellent results were obtained in 87% and 90% of patients respectively, however postoperative pH monitoring showed pathological reflux in 60% of patients after THM but in only 10% after a LHM with fundoplication [8]. The importance of fundoplication in limiting reflux in addition to myotomy was clearly shown by Richards and colleagues in 2004 [9]. In this prospective, randomized, double-blind clinical trial, patients with achalasia were assigned to undergo either Heller myotomy (21patients) or Heller myotomy plus Dor fundoplication (22 patients). Pathologic reflux (by pH monitoring) occurred in 10 of 21 patients (47.6%) after Heller and in 2 of 22 patients (9.1%) after Heller plus Dor ($p = 0.005$). No significant difference in outcome between the 2 techniques was observed with respect to postoperative lower-esophageal sphincter pressure or postoperative dysphagia score. Similar results have been recently documented by the group at the University of Padua, Italy [10]. Among 615 patients who underwent LHM with Dor fundoplication between 1992 and 2017, pathological reflux was identified by pH monitoring in 55 patients only (9.1%).

Technic of Laparoscopic Heller Myotomy and Dor Fundoplication

A liquid diet is recommended for at least 48 h before the operation because achalasia patients are at risk of aspiration during the anesthetic induction. Anesthesiologists should be aware of this risk and take appropriate precautions. The head of the bed must be elevated 30° until the airway is secured and a rapid sequence induction is recommended.

After endotracheal intubation, the patient is positioned supine in low lithotomy position over an inflated beanbag with the lower extremities extended on stirrups, with knees flexed 20°–30°. We routinely use pneumatic compression stockings to reduce the risk of deep vein thrombosis. The surgeon stands between the patient's legs, and the first and second assistants on the left and right side of the operating table, respectively.

- <u>Ports placement</u>

Five 10 mm ports are used for the operation. Port 1 is placed in the midline or slightly to the left about 14 cm below the xiphoid process. This port is used for insertion of the 30° scope. Ports 2 and 3 are placed about 2 cm below the right and left costal margins (forming an angle of about 120°). Port 4 is placed at the level of port 1 in the right mid-clavicular line (this is used for the liver retractor) and port 5 is placed at the level of port 1 in the left mid-clavicular line.

- Division of Gastrohepatic Ligament

Once the left segment of the liver is retracted and the gastroesophageal junction (GEJ) is adequately exposed, the gastrohepatic ligament is divided starting above the caudate lobe of the liver toward the right crus. The esophagus is then separated from the right crus using a hook cautery and blunt dissection. The posterior vagus nerve should be identified and preserved.

- Division of Phrenoesophageal Membrane

The phrenoesophageal membrane above the esophagus is divided. The anterior vagus is identified and left attached to the esophageal wall. The esophagus is then separated from the left pillar or the crus. If a Dor fundoplication is planned, the dissection is usually limited to the anterior and lateral aspects of the esophagus, and there is no need to perform a posterior dissection.

- Division of Short Gastric Vessels

Starting from a point midway along the greater curvature of the stomach, the short gastric vessels are taken down with a vessel sealing system all the way to the left pillar of the crus. This mobilization is important to avoid any tension when the Dor fundoplication is created.

- Esophageal Myotomy

The gastroesophageal fat pad should be dissected off the anterior surface of the stomach to expose the GEJ. The esophagus is pulled downward and to the left using a Babcock clamp applied over the junction. This maneuver will expose the right side of the esophagus. The myotomy is usually started about 3 cm above the GEJ at the 11 O′ clock position. Once the submucosal plane is identified, the myotomy is extended proximally for about 6 cm above the GEJ, and distally for about 2.5 cm onto the gastric wall for a total length of about 8–9 cm.

To perform the myotomy, we use a monopolar electrocautery with a 90° hook. Bleeding from the muscle edges should not be controlled with electrocautery but rather with compression with gauze to avoid injuring the esophageal mucosa. If an esophageal perforation occurs it should be repaired using 4-0 or 5-0 absorbable suture material.

- Dor Fundoplication

A partial fundoplication is performed to decrease the risk of postoperative reflux. The Dor fundoplication is an 180° anterior fundoplication that has two rows of sutures (left and right). The left row has three stitches: the uppermost stitch incorporates the fundus, the esophageal wall, and the left pillar of the crus; the other two incorporate the stomach and the cut edge of the myotomy. The gastric fundus is then folded over the exposed mucosa, placing the greater curvature next to the right pillar of the crus. The second row of stitches comprises three stitches between the fundus and the right pillar of the crus. Finally, we place two additional stitches between the superior edge of the fundoplication and the rim of the esophageal hiatus to avoid any tension created by the fundoplication.

Excellent results are also obtained when a Toupet fundoplication is used [11]. We do prefer a Dor fundoplication as it does not need a posterior dissection and because it covers the exposed mucosa. A Nissen fundoplication should be avoided as it determines a high resistance at the GEJ, causing recurrent dysphagia over time [12].

We do not routinely obtain a contrast study on postoperative day one. This is done only if a mucosal perforation occurred during the procedure to check the integrity of the repair. On postoperative day #1 patients are given a liquid diet for breakfast.

Most patients are discharged within 24 h and resume their regular activity within 2 weeks. Patients are instructed to avoid meat, carbonated drinks, and bread for 2 weeks.

The LHM has shown excellent results over the years. Costantini et al. showed that the outcome was excellent in 896 of 1001 patients (89.5%) at a median follow-up of 65 months [10]. The European multicenter study showed a success rate of 84% after 60 months [6]. The long-term results of a prospective and randomized trial in Sweden comparing PD and LHM showed that after LHM 92% of patients had excellent results after 5 years, and 80% at 10-year follow-up [13]. Based on these data, LHM with partial fundoplication is considered today the surgical procedure of choice in achalasia patients.

In our experience, the key elements of a successful operation are a myotomy extending on the gastric wall for about 2.5 cm and a partial fundoplication, either anterior or posterior.

Peroral Endoscopic Myotomy

In 2010 Dr. Inoue published the results of a new endoscopic technique called peroral endoscopic myotomy (POEM) for the treatment of esophageal achalasia, showing clinical success in 100% of seventeen patients with achalasia [1]. This initial report represents a milestone in the treatment of this disease, and today POEM is used in many centers across the world, either as primary treatment or for treating recurrent symptoms after pneumatic dilatation or LHM.

The procedure is usually done under general anesthesia and consists of 4 steps: (1) submucosal injection and mucosal incision, usually 10–12 cm above the GEJ; (2) submucosal tunneling, extended past the GEJ for 2–3 cm onto the stomach; (3) myotomy. The circular fibers are transected with preservation of the longitudinal fibers. The myotomy extends from 2 cm distal to the mucosal entry to 2–3 cm onto the gastric wall; and (4) closure of the mucosal entry with clips or endoscopic sutures.

Many studies have shown that POEM is effective in relieving symptoms in more than 90% of patients, suggesting that it might be considered the primary treatment modality for patients with achalasia. However, POEM has a clear "Achilles heel" due to a remarkably high incidence of post-procedure GERD, usually around 50%, as the procedure is based on a myotomy alone without a fundoplication. This finding reproduces the results of the prospective and randomized trial comparing a laparoscopic myotomy alone with a laparoscopic myotomy and Dor fundoplication that showed a 6-fold increase in pathologic reflux after a myotomy alone as compared to a myotomy and Dor fundoplication [9]. A meta-analysis by Schlottmann et al. comparing the efficacy of POEM and LHM and the incidence of post-procedure reflux in patients with achalasia, showed that control of symptoms was excellent with either procedure (at 2-year follow-up 92.7% after POEM and 90% after LHM). However, pH monitoring showed that the incidence of pathological reflux was more than 4-fold higher after POEM as compared to LHM with partial fundoplication (47.5% versus 11.1%) [14]. These findings have been recently confirmed in a multi-center, randomized, and controlled trial comparing the endoscopic and the surgical myotomy in patients with esophageal achalasia. A total of 221 patients were randomized to either POEM (112 patients) or LHM (109 patients) [15]. At 2-year follow-up clinical success was observed in 83% of patients in the POEM group and in 81.7% in the LHM group. The incidence of pathologic reflux was 57% after POEM and 20% after LHM.

This high incidence of GERD after POEM must be considered when treatment is chosen, particularly in young patients as a life-long exposure to reflux can cause esophagitis, strictures, Barrett's esophagus, and even adenocarcinoma.

The achalasia subtype, as shown by HRM, must be taken into consideration when planning treatment. Both LHM and POEM can be chosen as primary treatment for type I and II achalasia, but POEM is superior to LHM for type III, probably because it allows a longer myotomy onto the esophageal wall [16, 17].

Over the years we have developed the following treatment algorithm (Fig. 1), based on the data presented above our preferred initial treatment is a laparoscopic Heller myotomy with Dor fundoplication. If symptoms recur, we initially treat the patient with pneumatic dilatation as this approach has been shown to be safe and effective [18]. In case of failure of pneumatic dilatation, we use POEM, usually very safe as the myotomy can be done on the posterior wall of the esophagus [19]. Esophagectomy should be considered as a last resort only after the failure of all the other treatment modalities.

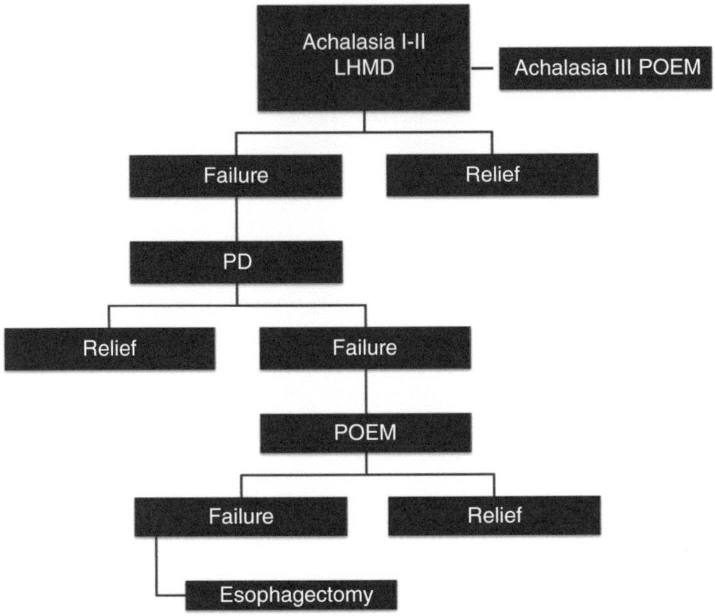

Fig. 1 Treatment algorithm of esophageal achalasia

Conclusions

Today we have 3 excellent treatment modalities to improve the quality of life of patients affected by achalasia. We feel that the best results are obtained in in multidisciplinary centers where expertise is present and the treatment can be tailored to the individual patient.

Conflict of Interest The Author has no conflict of interest to declare.

References

1. Inoue H, Minami H, Kobayashi Y, et al. Peroral endoscopic myotomy (POEM) for esophageal achalasia. Endoscopy. 2010;42:265–71.
2. Fisichella PM, Raz D, Palazzo F, Niponmick I, Patti MG. Clinical, radiological, and manometric profile in 145 patients with untreated achalasia. Word J Surg. 2008;32:1974–9.
3. Andolfi C, Kavitt RT, Herbella FA, Patti MG. Achalasia and respiratory symptoms. Effect of laparoscopic Heller myotomy. J Laparoendosc Adv Surg Tech A. 2016;26:675–9.
4. Yadlapati R, Kahrilas PJ, Fox MR, et al. Esophageal motility disorders on high resolution manometry: Chicago classification version 4.0. Neurogastroenterol Motil. 2021;33:1–36.
5. Boeckxstaens GE, Annese V, des Verannes SB, et al. Pneumatic dilation versus laparoscopic Heller's myotomy for idiopathic achalasia. N Engl J Med. 2011;364:1807–16.
6. Moonen A, Annese V, Belmans A, et al. Long-term results of the European achalasia trial: a multicentre randomized controlled trial comparing pneumatic dilation versus laparoscopic Heller myotomy. Gut. 2016;65:732–9.

7. Pellegrini C, Wetter LA, Patti M, et al. Thoracoscopic esophagomyotomy. Initial experience with a new approach for the treatment of achalasia. Ann Surg. 1992;216:291–6.
8. Patti MG, Arcerito M, De Pinto M, et al. Comparison of thoracoscopic and laparoscopic Heller myotomy for achalasia. J Gastrointest Surg. 1998;2:561–6.
9. Richards WO, Torquati A, Holzman MD, et al. Heller myotomy versus Heller myotomy with Dor fundoplication for achalasia: a prospective randomized double-blind clinical trial. Ann Surg. 2004;240:405–12.
10. Costantini M, Salvador R, Capovilla G, et al. A thousand and one laparoscopic Heller myotomies for esophageal achalasia: a 25-year experience at a single center. J Gastrointest Surg. 2019;23:23–35.
11. Alimi YR, Esquivel MM, Hawn MT. Laparoscopic Heller myotomy and Toupet fundoplication. World J Surg. 2022;46:1535–41.
12. Rebecchi F, Giaccone C, Farinella E, Campaci R, Morini M. Randomized controlled trial of laparoscopic Heller myotomy plus Dor fundoplication versus Nissen fundoplication for achalasia: long-term results. Ann Surg. 2008;248:1023–30.
13. Sediqi E, Tsoposidis A, Wallenius V, et al. Laparoscopic Heller myotomy or pneumatic dilatation in achalasia: results of a prospective, randomized study with at least a decade of follow-up. Surg Endosc. 2021;35:1618–25.
14. Schlottmann F, Luckett DJ, Fine J, Shaheen NJ, Patti MG. Laparoscopic Heller myotomy versus peroral endoscopic myotomy (POEM) for achalasia. A systematic review and meta-analysis. Ann Surg. 2018;267:451–60.
15. Werner YB, Hakanson B, Martinek J, et al. Endoscopic or surgical myotomy in patients with idiopathic achalasia. N Engl J Med. 2019;381:2219–29.
16. Kumbhari V, Tieu AH, Onimatu M, et al. Peroral endoscopic myotomy (POEM) vs laparoscopic Heller myotomy (LHM) for the treatment of type III achalasia in 75 patients: a multicenter comparative study. Endosc Int Open. 2015;3:195–201.
17. Sudashan M, Raja S, Adhikari S, et al. Peroral endoscopic myotomy provides effective palliation in type III achalasia. J Thorac Cardiovasc Surg. 2022;163:512–9.
18. Costantini A, Costantini M, Provenzano L, et al. Complimentary pneumatic dilations are an effective and safe treatment when laparoscopic myotomy fails. A 30-year experience at a single tertiary center. J Gastrointest Surg. 2024;28:1533–9.
19. Nabi Z, Ramchandani M, Basha J, et al. Peroral endoscopic myotomy in case with prior Heller myotomy. Outcomes at a median follow-up of 5 years. Gastroenterol Hepatol. 2023;38:2035–9.

Non-achalasia Esophageal Motility Disorders: Diagnosis and Treatment

Rafael C. Katayama, Fernando A. M. Herbella, Francisco Schlottmann, and Marco G. Patti

Introduction

Primary esophageal motility disorders (PEMD) are those named alterations in esophageal motility not attributed to an identifiable cause, such as gastroesophageal reflux disease (GERD) or opioid usage, e.g. [1]. They present with a specific manometric pattern. Thus, they may be considered diseases *per se*. PEMD classification evolved from the classical model proposed by Richter [2] in the beginning of the century, at the time of conventional manometry, to the Chicago Classification, now in its 4.0 version [3], adapted to the era of high-resolution manometry, and periodically updated by a panel of experts. Other tests, such as barium esophagram, do not define disease anymore but are only adjuvant tools for diagnosis confirmation.

Chicago classification brought new parameters and novel nomenclature to PEMD besides a hierarchical flow of diagnoses avoiding overlapping of diagnosis and prioritizing some findings over others. Accordingly, PEMD with altered relaxation of the lower esophageal sphincter (LES) has precedence over other diagnoses and peristalsis abnormalities have a determined rank (Fig. 1).

Among all PEMD, achalasia is certainly the only one with a reasonable consensus regarding diagnosis and treatment [4] and the one whose manometric definition has not changed along time.

R. C. Katayama · F. A. M. Herbella (✉)
Department of Surgery, Federal University of São Paulo, São Paulo, Brazil
e-mail: herbella.dcir@epm.br

F. Schlottmann
University of Buenos Aires, Ciudad Autónoma Buenos Aires, Buenos Aires, Argentina

M. G. Patti
Department of Surgery, University of Virginia Hospital, Charlottesville, VA, USA

F. Schlottmann et al. (eds.), *Esophageal Disorders*,
https://doi.org/10.1007/978-3-032-08179-7_12

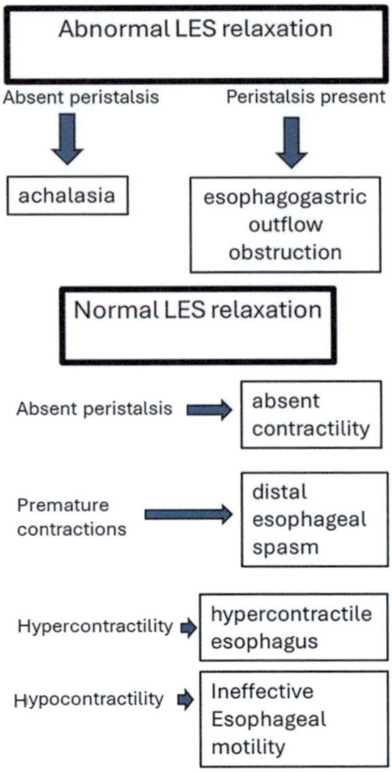

Fig. 1 Hierarchical flow of diagnoses for primary esophageal motility disorders based on high-resolution manometry findings according to the Chicago Classification 4.0 [3]. LES lower esophageal sphincter

Diagnosis

Esophagogastric Junction Outflow Obstruction

Esophagogastric junction outflow obstruction (EGJOO) is manometrically defined by "*abnormal median integrated relaxation pressure (IRP) (supine and upright), ≥20% elevated intrabolus pressure (supine), and not meeting criteria for achalasia*". In simpler and less technical words, manometry must show two characteristics. First, **abnormal relaxation of the LES**, as measured by the IRP, a complex parameter that calculates the mean pressure of 4 s of greatest post-deglutive relaxation in a 10 s gap, triggered at the beginning of a swallow, which corresponds to the relaxation of upper esophageal sphincter [5]. Second, **peristalsis preservation** to exclude the diagnosis of achalasia [6]. The presence of elevated intrabolus pressure confirms physiological obstruction. The current protocol demands confirmation of abnormal LES relaxation changing patient position during the test [7]. The protocol goes further suggesting pharmacological provocation with using amyl nitrite to confirm relaxation deficit [8] but this has not reached routine practice. Figure 2 illustrates a case of EGJOO.

Among the PEMD, EGJOO is probably the one that deserves more care to prevent overdiagnosis. Most cases are clinically irrelevant [3]. Thus, to be considered a disease, the manometric scenario must be accompanied by symptoms of

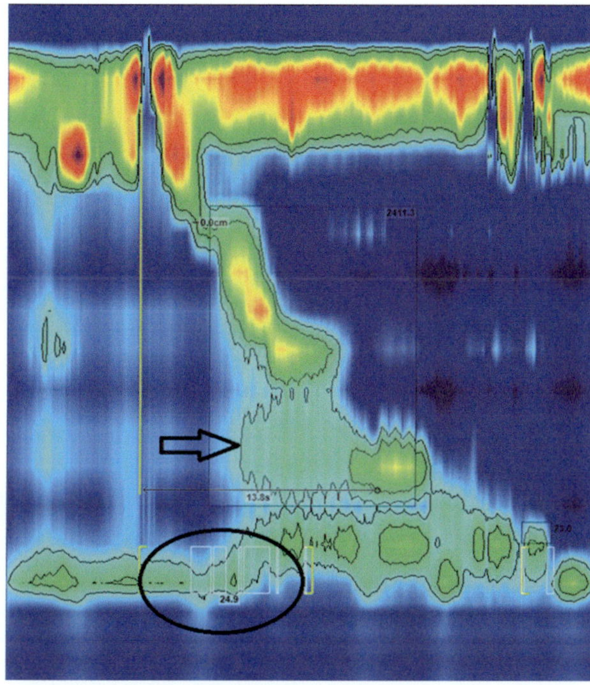

Fig. 2 Manometric tracing for esophagogastric junction outflow obstruction. Note abnormal LES relaxation during deglutition (circle), increased intrabolus pressure (arrow) and the presence of peristalsis

dysphagia and/or chest pain and confirmation with a supplementary test such as barium swallow or Functional Lumen Imaging Probe (FLIP) [3]. This is a frequent finding after operations at the esophagogastric junction [9] and in the presence of hiatal hernia [10].

Absent Contractility

Absent contractility is manometrically defined by *100% failed peristalsis with normal LES relaxation* (Fig. 3). Supportive tests may be used to rule out achalasia in dubious cases [11]. It is interesting that the current classification left the term aperistalsis to achalasia. This is frequently found in patients with diseases of the connective tissue affecting the esophagus and rarely in healthy volunteers.

Distal Esophageal Spasm

Distal esophageal spasm is manometrically defined by *≥20% swallows with premature/spastic contraction* [3] identified by a short distal latency parameter and normal LES relaxation (Fig. 4). Also here, to be considered a disease, the manometric scenario must be accompanied by symptoms of dysphagia and/or chest pain.

Fig. 3 Manometric tracing for absent contractility. Note peristalsis absence but normal lower esophageal sphincter relaxation

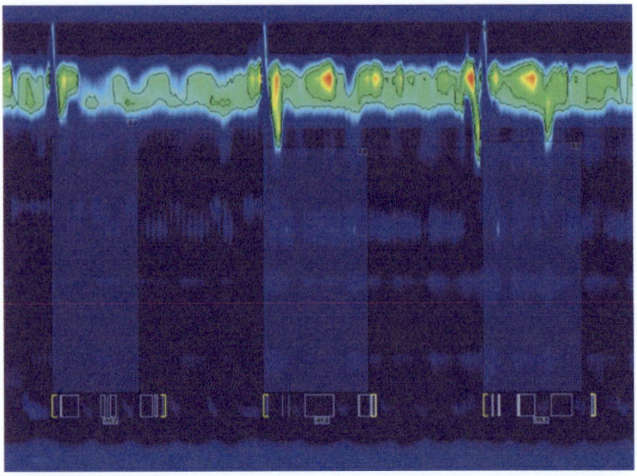

Fig. 4 Manometric tracing for distal esophageal spasm. Note premature waves shown as verticalized contractions (compare to normal wave in the inset)

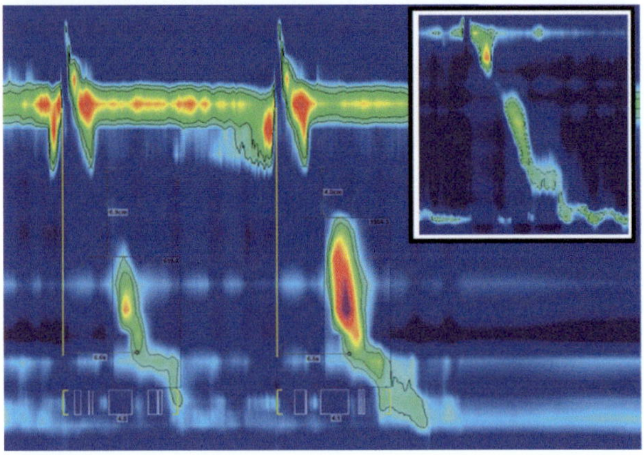

Hypercontractile Esophagus

Hypercontractile esophagus is manometrically defined by *≥20% hypercontractile swallows* and normal LES relaxation [12] (Fig. 5). This condition was previously called **nutcracker** esophagus during the conventional manometry era (some radiologists still use this nomenclature) and, posteriorly during the early high-resolution era, as **jackhammer** esophagus. Chicago Classification 4.0 defined subgroups for this condition, leaving the name jackhammer for a subset. This subclassification; however, is not much used due to the rarity of the disease, creating very small clusters if subgrouping is applied. Also here, to be considered a disease, the manometric scenario must be accompanied by symptoms of dysphagia and/or chest pain.

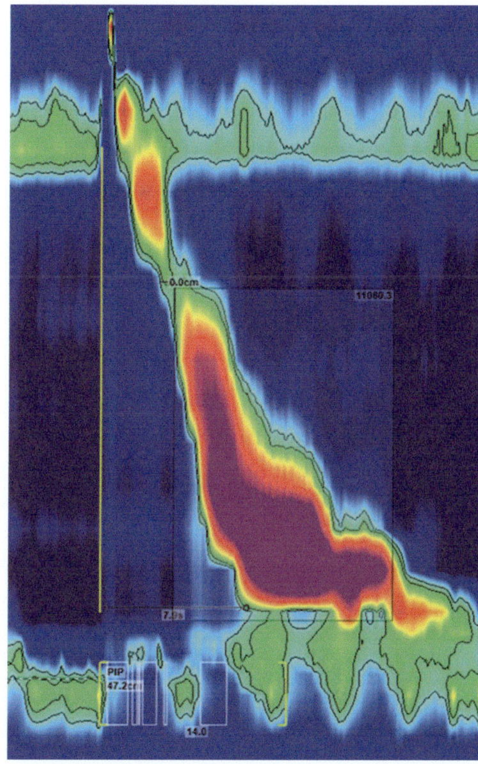

Fig. 5 Manometric tracing for hypercontractile esophagus. Note hypercontractile wave

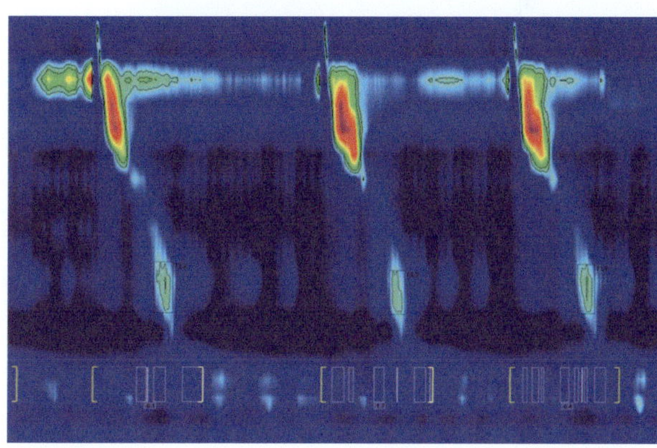

Fig. 6 Manometric tracing for ineffective esophageal motility. Note hypocontractile waves

Ineffective Esophageal Motility

Ineffective esophageal motility is manometrically defined by *>70% ineffective swallows* (weak contractions) *or ≥50% failed peristalsis* and normal LES relaxation [11] (Fig. 6). Some supportive tests are recommended in dubious cases but with a low degree of evidence: poor bolus transit on impedance or barium esophagram and lack of contraction reserve on the provocative test of multiple rapid swallows [3].

Treatment

Esophagogastric Junction Outflow Obstruction

As above mentioned, most EGJOO cases are secondary to mechanical obstruction or operations at the esophagogastric junction. These cases should be treated accordingly, and they will not be discussed in this chapter. EGJOO as a PEMD represents a functional obstacle at the esophagogastric junction similar to achalasia. As such, therapy is aimed towards destroying the LES either by endoscopic pneumatic dilatation, peroral endoscopic myotomy (POEM) or Heller's myotomy and fundoplication. However, if symptoms are mild, it is licit to adopt a conservative wait-and-see management since spontaneous resolution of symptoms over 6 months is possible in up to ¾ of the patients [13]. Pharmacological therapy, on the other hand, shows variable, usually bad and short-duration outcomes [13].

Pneumatic dilatation has been tried in the setting of EGJOO. Most series encompass a small number of patients (frequently below 30) with 30–70% symptom resolution [14–16]. Unfortunately, there are no studies with post-procedure pHmonitoring, since GERD is the main drawback of the method, as shown by the experience gathered with achalasia treatment. Cases treated by Heller's myotomy showed good outcomes while POEM did not show good results at the beginning of experience [17]. Currently both treatments are comparable, with symptoms resolution in over 80% of the cases, even though POEM has a higher incidence of GERD [18], again, following the same experience as found for achalasia.

Absent Contractility

Absent contractility is a rare finding as a PEMD, i.e., in the absence of opioid usage or connective tissue diseases. Absent contractility in the setting of connective tissue diseases is frequently associated with GERD and therapy should be aimed at GERD [19]. Most cases therapy is limited to lifestyle and dietetic modification with some attempts to use prokinetics drugs but mostly not successful [20].

Some isolated reports advocate achalasia-like treatment aimed at the LES ion selected cases where functional obstruction at the esophagogastric junction can be demonstrated [21, 22].

Distal Esophageal Spasm

Distal esophageal spasm and hypercontractile esophagus are frequently grouped as *spastic disorders of motility*. Therapy is aimed towards decreasing muscular contraction, this time not only of the LES, but of the esophageal body.

Medical treatment mostly targets symptomatic relief and often fails [23]. There are no studies on Heller's myotomy for distal esophageal spasm based on the current classification. Previously, lack of LES relaxation could be part of the disease, and most series aimed at these patients. Current classification would include these cases as EGJOO. Some case reports of POEM for distal spasm have been reported with some multicenter studies but never surpassing 20 patients [17]. Results seem to be promising in selected patients [23].

Hypercontractile Esophagus

Just like distal esophageal spasm, therapy is aimed towards decreasing muscular contraction, this time not only of the LES, but of the esophageal body. Also, similar to distal spasm, current definition precludes a lack of relaxation of the LES, thus old literature should be viewed with discretion.

There are few studies based on the new classification. Even worse, some mix results for different PEMD and include patients with GERD [24].

There are no studies with Heller's myotomy. POEM has been only evaluated in a few uncontrolled studies in small cohorts [25]. Results are good in these series with symptom control in over 80% of the cases [25–27], data supported by a recent meta-analysis [28].

Ineffective Esophageal Motility

The treatment for ineffective esophageal motility is similar to absent contractility. Pharmacological therapy is more a future perspective than a clinical reality [29]. Most cases therapy is limited to lifestyle and dietetic modification. We have routinely referred patients with primary IEM and dysphagia to speech language therapy and satisfaction has been consistently good. Speech language therapists are able to teach forceful swallow maneuvers using the pharyngeal pump to help esophageal peristalsis, probably very similar to achalasia patients [30]. Also, they may rehabilitate swallow practices such as rapid eating [31].

Conclusion

PEMD presents with unique manometric patterns. Thus, diagnosis is dependent and exclusive of esophageal manometry. Adjunct tests can and should be used in dubious cases or to provide confirmation of the diagnosis. GERD, and less frequently other causes as well, may be the causative factor for most manometric patterns that define the PEMDs. Symptoms are not discriminatory [32], thus pHmonitoring is also essential in the workup of these patients. If GERD is present, therapy is aimed at reflux control.

Treatment is usually aimed towards actions modulating esophageal contractions for the spastic disorders and lifestyle changes for the hypomotilities.

Conflict of Interest The authors have no conflict of interest.

References

1. Herbella FA, Raz DJ, Nipomnick I, Patti MG. Primary versus secondary esophageal motility disorders: diagnosis and implications for treatment. J Laparoendosc Adv Surg Tech A. 2009;19(2):195–8. https://doi.org/10.1089/lap.2008.0317.
2. Richter JE. Oesophageal motility disorders. Lancet. 2001;358(9284):823–8. https://doi.org/10.1016/S0140-6736(01)05973-6.
3. Yadlapati R, Kahrilas PJ, Fox MR, Bredenoord AJ, Prakash Gyawali C, Roman S, Babaei A, Mittal RK, Rommel N, Savarino E, Sifrim D, Smout A, Vaezi MF, Zerbib F, Akiyama J, Bhatia S, Bor S, Carlson DA, Chen JW, Cisternas D, Cock C, Coss-Adame E, de Bortoli N, Defilippi C, Fass R, Ghoshal UC, Gonlachanvit S, Hani A, Hebbard GS, Wook Jung K, Katz P, Katzka DA, Khan A, Kohn GP, Lazarescu A, Lengliner J, Mittal SK, Omari T, Park MI, Penagini R, Pohl D, Richter JE, Serra J, Sweis R, Tack J, Tatum RP, Tutuian R, Vela MF, Wong RK, Wu JC, Xiao Y, Pandolfino JE. Esophageal motility disorders on high-resolution manometry: Chicago classification version 4.0©. Neurogastroenterol Motil. 2021;33(1):e14058. https://doi.org/10.1111/nmo.14058. Erratum in: Neurogastroenterol Motil. 2024;36(2):e14179. doi: 10.1111/nmo.14179.
4. Patti MG, Herbella FA. Achalasia and other esophageal motility disorders. J Gastrointest Surg. 2011;15(5):703–7. https://doi.org/10.1007/s11605-011-1478-x.
5. Lafraia FM, Herbella FAM, Kalluf JR, Patti MG. A pictorial presentation of Esophageal high resolution Manometry current parameters. Arq Bras Cir Dig. 2017;30(1):69–71. https://doi.org/10.1590/0102-6720201700010019.
6. Herbella FA, Armijo PR, Patti MG. A pictorial presentation of 3.0 Chicago Classification for esophageal motility disorders. Einstein (Sao Paulo). 2016;14(3):439–42. https://doi.org/10.1590/S1679-45082016MD3444.
7. Fox MR, Sweis R, Yadlapati R, Pandolfino J, Hani A, Defilippi C, Jan T, Rommel N. Chicago classification version 4.0© technical review: update on standard high-resolution manometry protocol for the assessment of esophageal motility. Neurogastroenterol Motil. 2021;33(4):e14120. https://doi.org/10.1111/nmo.14120.
8. Babaei A, Shad S, Szabo A, Massey BT. Pharmacologic interrogation of patients with esophagogastric junction outflow obstruction using amyl nitrite. Neurogastroenterol Motil. 2019;31(9):e13668. https://doi.org/10.1111/nmo.13668.
9. Wilshire CL, Niebisch S, Watson TJ, Litle VR, Peyre CG, Jones CE, Peters JH. Dysphagia postfundoplication: more commonly hiatal outflow resistance than poor esophageal body motility. Surgery. 2012;152(4):584–92; discussion 592-4. https://doi.org/10.1016/j.surg.2012.07.014.
10. Herbella FAM, Patti MG, Filho RM, et al. How changes in treatment guidelines affect the standard of care: ethical opinions using the Chicago 4.0 Classification for Esophageal motility disorders as example. Foregut. 2022;2(2):111–5. https://doi.org/10.1177/26345161221081038.
11. Gyawali CP, Zerbib F, Bhatia S, Cisternas D, Coss-Adame E, Lazarescu A, Pohl D, Yadlapati R, Penagini R, Pandolfino J. Chicago Classification update (V4.0): technical review on diagnostic criteria for ineffective esophageal motility and absent contractility. Neurogastroenterol Motil. 2021;33(8):e14134. https://doi.org/10.1111/nmo.14134.
12. Chen JW, Savarino E, Smout A, Xiao Y, de Bortoli N, Yadlapati R, Cock C. Chicago Classification Update (v4.0): technical review on diagnostic criteria for hypercontractile esophagus. Neurogastroenterol Motil. 2021;33(6):e14115. https://doi.org/10.1111/nmo.14115.
13. Beveridge C, Lynch K. Diagnosis and Management of Esophagogastric Junction Outflow Obstruction. Gastroenterol Hepatol (N Y). 2020;16(3):131–8.
14. Desai N, Kline M, Duncan D, Godiers M, Patel V, Keilin S, Jain AS. Expanding the role of pneumatic dilation for nonachalasia patients: a comparative study. Gastrointest Endosc. 2023;97(2):251–9. https://doi.org/10.1016/j.gie.2022.09.032.
15. Sloan JA, Triggs JR, Pandolfino JE, Dbouk M, Brewer Gutierrez OI, El Zein M, Quader F, Ichkhanian Y, Gyawali CP, Rubenstein JH, Khashab MA. Treatment experience with a novel 30-mm hydrostatic balloon in esophageal dysmotility: a multicenter retrospective analysis. Gastrointest Endosc. 2020;92(6):1251–7. https://doi.org/10.1016/j.gie.2020.04.076.

16. Clayton SB, Shin CM, Ewing A, Blonski W, Richter J. Pneumatic dilation improves esophageal emptying and symptoms in patients with idiopathic esophago-gastric junction outflow obstruction. Neurogastroenterol Motil. 2019;31(3):e13522. https://doi.org/10.1111/nmo.13522.
17. Herbella FAM, Schlottmann F. Minimally invasive surgery for non-achalasia primary esophageal motility disorders is currently underused. Mini-invasive Surg. 2019;3:24. https://doi.org/10.20517/2574-1225.2019.20.
18. Sarici IS, Eriksson S, Abu-Nuwar MR, Kuzy J, Gardner M, Zheng P, Jobe B, Ayazi S. Peroral Endoscopic Myotomy (POEM) and laparoscopic Heller Myotomy with Dor Fundoplication for Esophagogastric Junction Outflow Obstruction (EGJOO): a comparison of outcomes and impact on physiology. J Gastrointest Surg. 2023;27(11):2684–93. https://doi.org/10.1007/s11605-023-05844-0.
19. Menezes MA, Herbella FA, Patti MG. Laparoscopic Antireflux surgery in patients with connective tissue diseases. J Laparoendosc Adv Surg Tech A. 2016;26(4):296–8. https://doi.org/10.1089/lap.2016.0097.
20. Patel DA, Yadlapati R, Vaezi MF. Esophageal motility disorders: current approach to diagnostics and therapeutics. Gastroenterology. 2022;162(6):1617–34. https://doi.org/10.1053/j.gastro.2021.12.289.
21. Zhao Q, Chen P, Wang X, Ye H, Zhang X, Song Y, Zhang X. Is Peroral endoscopic Myotomy a potential therapy for Esophageal absent contractility? Surg Laparosc Endosc Percutan Tech. 2020;30(2):129–33. https://doi.org/10.1097/SLE.0000000000000770.
22. Cohen DL, Bermont A, Richter V, Azzam N, Shirin H, Dickman R, Mari A. Integrated Relaxation Pressure (IRP) distinguishes between reflux-predominant and dysphagia-predominant phenotypes of Esophageal "Absent Contractility". J Clin Med. 2022;11(21):6287. https://doi.org/10.3390/jcm11216287.
23. Gorti H, Samo S, Shahnavaz N, Qayed E. Distal esophageal spasm: update on diagnosis and management in the era of high-resolution manometry. World J Clin Cases. 2020;8(6):1026–32. https://doi.org/10.12998/wjcc.v8.i6.1026.
24. Chandan S, Mohan BP, Chandan OC, Jha LK, Mashiana HS, et al. Clinical efficacy of per-oral endoscopic myotomy (POEM) for spastic esophageal disorders: a systematic review and meta-analysis. Surg Endosc. 2019; https://doi.org/10.1007/s00464-019-06819-6.
25. Savarino E, Smout AJPM. The hypercontractile esophagus: still a tough nut to crack. Neurogastroenterol Motil. 2020;32(11):e14010. https://doi.org/10.1111/nmo.14010.
26. Canakis A, Xie G, Kim RE. Peroral endoscopic Myotomy is an effective treatment option for managing Jackhammer Esophagus: a single center experience. J Clin Gastroenterol. 2023;57(6):569–73. https://doi.org/10.1097/MCG.0000000000001717.
27. Morley TJ, Mikulski MF, Rade M, Chalhoub J, Desilets DJ, Romanelli JR. Per-oral endoscopic myotomy for the treatment of non-achalasia esophageal dysmotility disorders: experience from a single high-volume center. Surg Endosc. 2023;37(2):1013–20. https://doi.org/10.1007/s00464-022-09596-x.
28. Puri R, Giri S, Panigrahi SC, Mallick B, Nath P, Sharma ZD, Sahu BK. Efficacy and safety of per-oral endoscopic myotomy in non-achalasia esophageal motility disorders: a systematic review and meta-analysis. Esophagus. 2024;21(4):419–29. https://doi.org/10.1007/s10388-024-01076-6.
29. Jandee S, Geeraerts A, Geysen H, Rommel N, Tack J, Vanuytsel T. Management of Ineffective Esophageal Hypomotility. Front Pharmacol. 2021;12:638915. https://doi.org/10.3389/fphar.2021.638915.
30. Menezes MA, Herbella FA, Patti MG. High-resolution Manometry evaluation of the Pharynx and upper Esophageal Sphincter motility in patients with Achalasia. J Gastrointest Surg. 2015;19(10):1753–7. https://doi.org/10.1007/s11605-015-2901-5.
31. Li KL, Chen JH, Zhang Q, Huizinga JD, Vadakepeedika S, Zhao YR, Yu WZ, Luo HS. Habitual rapid food intake and ineffective esophageal motility. World J Gastroenterol. 2013;19(14):2270–7. https://doi.org/10.3748/wjg.v19.i14.2270.
32. de Padua F, Herbella FAM, Patti MG. The prevalence of gastroesophageal reflux disease in named manometric patterns of dysmotility according to the Chicago Classification 4.0. Dis Esophagus. 2022;35(10):doac023. https://doi.org/10.1093/dote/doac023.

Epiphrenic Diverticulum

Fernando A. M. Herbella, Francisco Schlottmann, and Marco G. Patti

Epiphrenic diverticulum (ED) is a pulsion diverticulum located in the distal 10 cm of the esophagus. It is due to the herniation of the mucosa and submucosa through the muscle layers of the esophageal wall.

Pathophysiology

While initially it was thought that an ED was a primary anatomic abnormality, more than 60 years ago Effler and Belsey suggested that an ED was probably secondary to an underlying esophageal motility disorder [1, 2]. However, even today, this issue is still controversial. Some authors, in fact, feel that a primary motility disorder such as achalasia underlies the development of the diverticulum in 75%–100% of cases [3, 4], while others believe that this relationship is not as frequent [5, 6]. The implications are very important as to whether a myotomy should be a routine part of the operation instead of being used in selected cases.

Achalasia and diffuse esophageal spasm are the disorders more commonly documented. A possible explanation for the finding of normal motility by manometry in some patients may be due to the intermittent nature of diffuse esophageal spasm. During a conventional manometry, lower esophageal sphincter function and esophageal peristalsis are usually assessed by observing ten swallows of 5 ml of water at 30 s intervals. Therefore, it is possible that during the 30–40 s of the test, spastic activity is not present. The hypothesis that a primary esophageal motility disorder is

F. A. M. Herbella
Department of Surgery, Federal University of São Paulo, São Paulo, São Paulo, Brazil

F. Schlottmann
University of Buenos Aires, Ciudad Autónoma Buenos Aires, Buenos Aires, Argentina

M. G. Patti (✉)
Department of Surgery, University of Virginia Hospital, Charlottesville, VA, USA

F. Schlottmann et al. (eds.), *Esophageal Disorders*,
https://doi.org/10.1007/978-3-032-08179-7_13

present in all patients with ED was tested by Nehra and colleagues using ambulatory manometry (which allows the analysis of 1000 swallows over 24 h), in addition to standard manometry [3]. Among 21 patients with ED, an esophageal disorder was demonstrated in 71% of patients by standard manometry but in 100% of patients when the ambulatory test was used. The findings of this study are very important as they support the routine performance of a myotomy regardless of the findings of the standard esophageal manometry.

Clinical Presentation

Dysphagia, regurgitation, chest pain and weight loss are the most common symptoms. These symptoms are thought to be secondary to the underlying motility disorder rather than the diverticulum [7]. Heartburn can be present, and it is secondary to stasis and fermentation of the retained food rather than real gastroesophageal reflux. Some patients can present with respiratory symptoms such as cough, asthma, and pneumonia [8]. Complications such as bleeding and perforation are rare [9, 10]. The development of a squamous cell carcinoma within the diverticulum has been reported and stresses the importance of endoscopic follow-up in patients with an untreated asymptomatic diverticulum or when a myotomy alone is performed leaving the diverticulum in place [11].

Evaluation

Barium Swallow The barium swallow is probably the most important test for establishing the diagnosis and for planning the operation. This test defines the location of the ED (right or left), the size of the neck, and the distance from the gastroesophageal junction (Fig. 1).

In 70%–75% of patients the diverticulum is located on the right side [8] and 10%–15% of patients have two or more diverticula [12].

Endoscopy Because dysphagia is often the presenting symptom, endoscopy is necessary to rule out cancer. In addition, when the manometry catheter does not cross the gastroesophageal junction, endoscopy under sedation allows proper placement of the catheter [13].

Esophageal Manometry Standard manometry identifies associated motility disorders in 70%–85% of patients. Based on the data available, and our own experience [8], it seems that this test is often of academic interest but does not affect management when a myotomy is routinely included.

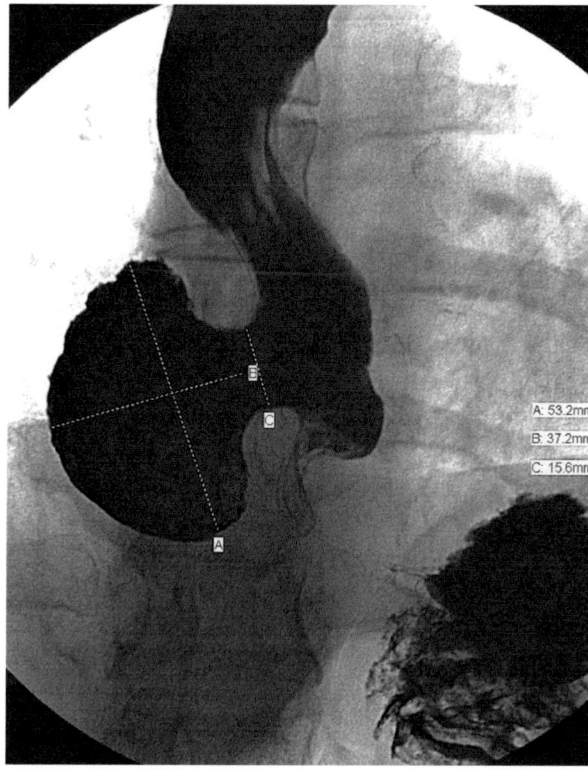

Fig. 1 Barium swallow with measurement of size of the pouch, size of the neck and distance from the gastroesophageal junction

Treatment

Indications We and others believe that treatment should be reserved for symptomatic patients only. This approach is based on two reasons: (1) fewer than 10% of asymptomatic patients develop symptoms due to the diverticulum [14]; and (2) even in expert hands the operation carries significant morbidity and mortality [15, 16].

In some patients the diverticulum is an incidental finding on a chest X-ray. However, before classifying these diverticula as "asymptomatic", it is important to evaluate for the presence not only of esophageal symptoms such as dysphagia or regurgitation, but also for respiratory symptoms such as night cough, asthma, or pneumonia which might be due to aspiration and lead to severe complications [17].

Laparoscopic Diverticulectomy, Myotomy and Dor Fundoplication

The initial steps (port placement, division of the gastrohepatic ligament, division of the phrenoesophageal membrane, and division of the short gastric vessels) are like those of a laparoscopic Heller myotomy for patients with achalasia [18].

Dissection It can be very demanding especially for higher diverticula. The most challenging aspect is the identification of the upper border of the diverticulum and of its neck. It is important to dissect the neck of the diverticulum free of the surrounding tissue and clearly identify the muscle layers before the stapler is applied. We find it very useful to pass a Penrose drain around the gastroesophageal junction as it allows traction facilitating the dissection in the posterior mediastinum.

Transection of the diverticulum After the entire diverticulum is freed from surrounding structures and the neck is clearly identified, a 50-F to 56-F bougie is placed inside the esophagus to avoid narrowing of the lumen when the stapler is applied. A reticulating stapler is placed across the diverticular neck, parallel to the esophageal body, and the height of the staples is based on the thickness of the tissue at the transection site. Depending on the size of the neck, more than one application might be necessary. After inspection for staple line formation and bleeding, the muscle layers are approximated over the staple line using interrupted sutures.

Myotomy The myotomy should be done 180° opposite the diverticulum to avoid interference with the muscle closure. The myotomy should extend upward all the way to the diverticular neck and downward for about 2.5 cm onto the gastric wall.

Closure of the esophageal hiatus As the esophageal hiatus is quite wide at the end of the dissection, the crura should be approximated before the fundoplication is performed.

Partial fundoplication Because of the abnormal esophageal peristalsis, it is felt that a total fundoplication can create too much resistance at the level of the gastroesophageal junction, so that most authors prefer either a Dor or a Toupet fundoplication [18–20]. While in patients with achalasia a total fundoplication can cause recurrence of symptoms over time [21], in patients with achalasia and ED it can also cause a leak from the staple line because of the high intraluminal pressure [16].

The Evolution of the Treatment of Epiphrenic Diverticulum

Two considerations question the wisdom of resecting the diverticulum in addition to the myotomy and fundoplication: (1) most symptoms are caused by the underlying esophageal motility disorder rather than the diverticulum per se; and (2) the diverticulectomy is the component of the operation that is most frequently the cause of morbidity and mortality secondary to a leak from the staple line [16, 22]. Specifically, would a myotomy alone without diverticulectomy ameliorate the symptoms experienced by the patients?

A very important study addressing this question was published by Allaix and colleagues from the University of Chicago [7]. They compared the outcome of six patients with ED who underwent myotomy, diverticulectomy and Dor fundoplication to that of seven patients in whom the diverticulum was left in place, because very small in 3 (between 2 and 3 cm) or for technical reasons in four patients (the upper pole of the diverticulum and the neck could not be safely dissected because of severe adhesions or because too far from the gastroesophageal junction) (Fig. 2). Both the duration of symptoms (36 ± 33 vs. 30 ± 35 months) and the Eckardt score (6.5 ± 2.1 vs. 6.6 ± 3.3) were similar in the two groups. One patient in the diverticulectomy group had a staple line leak that was successfully treated by a combination of a drain placed by interventional radiology, next to the staple line, total parental nutrition, and endoscopic clips (Figs. 3 and 4). The study showed a similar resolution of symptoms in the two groups: at a median follow-up of 2 years the Eckardt score was 0 in the excised ED group and 0.1 in the non-excised group [23].

Wescott and colleagues recently described the result of the "myotomy first approach" in 22 patients with ED [23]. There were no perioperative complications, and the average length of stay was 2.5 days. At a mean follow-up of 68 months, dysphagia was resolved in 77% and regurgitation in 86% of patients. Three patients had persistent symptoms and two of them underwent a transthoracic diverticulectomy (one patient with resolution of symptoms and one patient with no improvement).

Based on the prior considerations and the results of these studies showing that in most patients the diverticulum can be left in place without sequelae, peroral

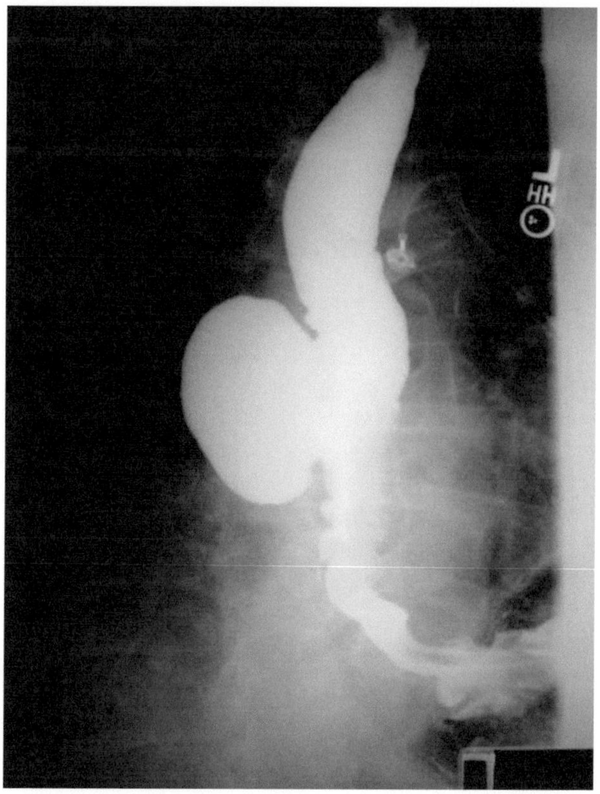

Fig. 2 Barium swallow shows a right-side diverticulum in a patient with diffuse esophageal spasm. Because of the distance from the gastroesophageal junction, it was left in place and a myotomy and Dor fundoplication were performed. The patient had complete resolution of dysphagia and regurgitation

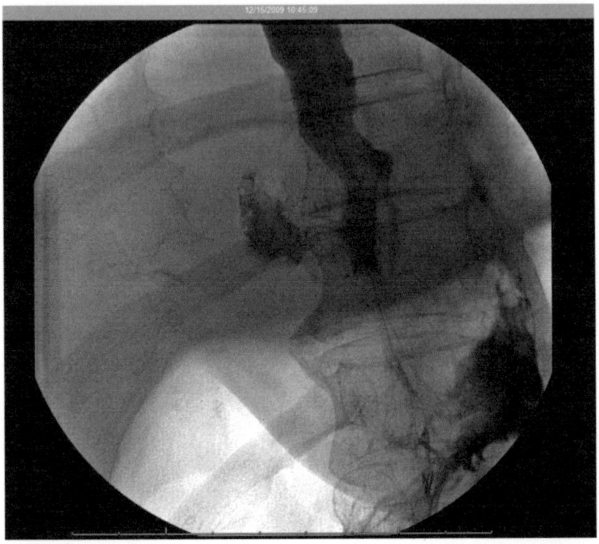

Fig. 3 Esophageal leak from the staple line

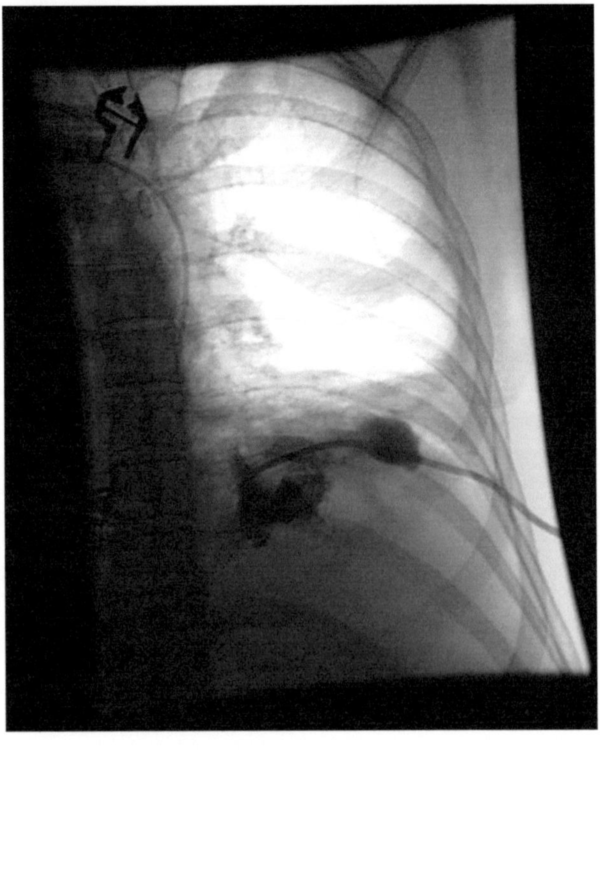

Fig. 4 Percutaneous drainage of esophageal leak

endoscopic myotomy (POEM) has been recently used successfully for the treatment of ED [24–28].

A recent international multicenter study evaluated the clinical outcome of POEM with and without septotomy in patients with symptomatic ED [28]. A total of 85 patients were treated in 21 centers between January 2014 and January 2023. The most common underlying disorder was achalasia. Clinical success was defined as Eckardt score < 3, or 1 point drop in the score for patients with baseline score <3, without the need for repeat surgical or endoscopic intervention during follow-up. At a median follow-up of 8 months, clinical success was excellent and similar in the two groups (POEM and septotomy 89.6% with Eckardt score of 1—POEM alone in 89.2% with Eckardt score of 1). A leak occurred in one patient (1.2%, managed with antibiotics, chest tubes and endoscopic treatment), and two patients had bleeding (managed with blood transfusions and endoscopic treatment). Reflux symptoms occurred in 26.5% of patients and endoscopy showed esophagitis in 21.3% of them. Fifty-three per cent of patients were taking PPI medications. This study clearly shows that POEM has a role in the treatment of patients with ED as it is technically feasible and safe, with excellent short-term clinical outcomes, and has the advantage of allowing a longer myotomy while being less invasive than surgery. However, as shown in achalasia patients treated with POEM, it is associated with a much higher rate of pathologic reflux as compared with a laparoscopic Heller myotomy with fundoplication [29, 30].

Overall, we feel that because ED is a very rare disorder, patients should be treated in a multidisciplinary center where therapy can be tailored to the individual patient and complications treated successfully.

Conflict of Interest The Author has no conflict of interest to declare.

References

1. Effler DB, Barr D, Groves LK. Epiphrenic diverticulum of the esophagus: surgical treatment. Arch Surg. 1959;79:459–67.
2. Belsey R. Functional disease of the esophagus. J Thorac Cardiovasc Surg. 1966;52:164–88.
3. Nehra D, Lord RV, DeMeester TR, et al. Physiologic basis for the treatment of epiphrenic diverticulum. Ann Surg. 2002;235:346–54.
4. Melman L, Quinlan J, Robertson B, et al. Esophageal manometric characteristics and outcomes for laparoscopic esophageal diverticulectomy, myotomy, and partial fundoplication for epiphrenic diverticula. Surg Endosc. 2009;23:1337–41.
5. Benacci JC, Deschamps C, Trastek VF, et al. Epiphrenic diverticulum: results of surgical treatment. Ann Thorac Surg. 1993;55:1109–13.
6. Streitz JM, Glick ME, Ellis FH. Selective use of myotomy for treatment of epiphrenic diverticula. Manometric and clinical analysis. Arch Surg. 1992;127:585–7.
7. Allaix ME, Borraez Segura BA, Herbella FA, Fisichella PM, Patti MG. Is resection of an esophageal epiphrenic diverticulum always necessary in the setting of achalasia? World J Surg. 2015;39:203–7.
8. Tedesco P, Fisichella PM, Way LW, Patti MG. Cause and treatment of epiphrenic diverticula. Am J Surg. 2005;190:902–5.

9. Abul-Khair MH, Khalil A, Mohsen A. Bleeding from an epiphrenic oesophageal diverticulum. Eur J Surg. 1992;158:377–8.
10. Ju-Hyeon L, Hiun-Suk C, Kwan-Hyoung K, et al. Delayed primary repair of perforated epiphrenic diverticulum. J Korean Med Sci. 2004;19:887–90.
11. Yoshida T, Hashimoto S, Mizuno KI, et al. Advanced squamous cell carcinoma in an asymptomatic, large, epiphrenic esophageal diverticulum. Clin J Gastroenterol. 2020;13:477–82.
12. Fasano NC, Levine MS, Rubesin SE, et al. Epiphrenic diverticulum: clinical and radiographic findings in 27 patients. Dysphagia. 2003;18:9–15.
13. Cohen DL, Bermont A, Richter V, et al. Technical success in performing esophageal high-resolution manometry in patients with an epiphrenic diverticulum. Dysphagia. 2024;39:282–8.
14. Zaninotto G, Portale G, Costantini M, et al. Therapeutic strategies for epiphrenic diverticula: systematic review. World J Surg. 2011;35:1447–53.
15. Zaninotto G, Portale G, Costantini M, et al. Long-term outcome of operated and non-operated epiphrenic diverticula. J Gastrointest Surg. 2008;12:1485–90.
16. Rossetti G, Fei L, del Genio G, et al. Epiphrenic diverticula minimally invasive surgery: a challenge for expert surgeons. Personal experience and review of the literature. Scand J Surg. 2013;102:129–35.
17. Debas HT, Payne WS, Cameron AJ, Carlson HC. Physiopathology of lower esophageal diverticulum and its implications for treatment. Surg Gynecol Obstet. 1980;151:593–600.
18. Orlow R, Herbella FA, Patti MG. Laparoscopic Heller myotomy with Dor fundoplication: an operation that has withstood the test of time. World J Surg. 2022;46:1531–4.
19. Soares RV, Montenovo M, Pellegrini CA, Oelschlager BK. Laparoscopy as the initial approach for epiphrenic diverticula. Surg Endosc. 2011;25:3740–6.
20. Patti MG, Herbella FA. Fundoplication after laparoscopic Heller myotomy for esophageal achalasia. What type? J Gastrointest Surg. 2010;14:1453–88.
21. Rebecchi F, Giaccone C, Farinella E, Campaci R, Morino M. Randomized controlled trial of laparoscopic Heller myotomy plus Dor fundoplication versus Nissen fundoplication for achalasia: long-term results. Ann Surg. 2008;248:1023–30.
22. Fernando HC, Luketich JD, Samphire J, et al. Minimally invasive operation for esophageal diverticula. Ann Thorac Surg. 2005;80:2076–81.
23. Westcott CJ, O'Connor S, Preiss JE, Patti MG, Farrell TM. Myotomy-first approach to epiphrenic esophageal diverticula. J Laparoendosc Adv Surg Tech A. 2019;29:726–9.
24. Kinoshita M, Tanaka S, Kawara F, et al. Peroral endoscopic myotomy alone is effective for esophageal motility disorders and esophageal epiphrenic diverticulum: a retrospective single-center study. Surg Endosc. 2020;34:5447–54.
25. Basile P, Gonzales JM, Le Mouel JP, et al. Per-oral endoscopic myotomy with septotomy for the treatment of distal esophageal diverticula (D-POEM). Surg Endosc. 2020;34:2321–5.
26. Samanta J, Mandavdhare HS, Kumar N, et al. Per-oral endoscopic myotomy for the management of large esophageal diverticula (D-POEM): safe and effective modality for complete septotomy. Dysphagia. 2022;37:84–92.
27. Wessels EM, Schultenmaker JM, Bastlaansen BAJ, et al. Efficacy and safety of peroral endoscopic myotomy for esophageal diverticula. Endosc Int Open. 2023;11:546–52.
28. Shrigiriwar A, Mony S, Fayyaz F, et al. Clinical outcomes of peroral endoscopic myotomy with and without septotomy for management of epiphrenic diverticula: an international multicenter experience. Gastrointest Endosc. 2024;100:840–8.
29. Schlottmann F, Luckett DJ, Shaheen NJ, Patti MG. Laparoscopic Heller myotomy versus peroral endoscopic myotomy (POEM) for achalasia. A systematic review and meta-analysis. Ann Surg. 2018;267:451–60.
30. Sanaka MR, Thota PN, Parikh MP, et al. Peropral endoscopic myotomy leads to higher rates of abnormal esophageal acid exposure tha laparoscopic Heller myotomy in achalasia. Surg Endosc. 2019;33:2284–92.

Eosinophilic Esophagitis

Jeremy A. Klein and Robert T. Kavitt

Epidemiology

EoE was first reported in the literature in 1978 and has been increasingly recognized in both pediatric and adult populations [1]. Population-based studies of EoE epidemiology show large heterogeneity based on study methodology and geographic location [2]. A 2022 meta-analysis estimated a worldwide pooled incidence of 5.31 per 100,000 person-years and a pooled prevalence of 40.04 cases per 100,000 person-years [3]. Both incidence and prevalence were noted to be higher in adults than in children. In adults, the disorder is most commonly diagnosed during the third decade of life [4, 5]. Other studies have found prevalence to be as high as 56.7 per 100,000 persons in the United States, equivalent to 152,152 cases [6]. Men are more commonly affected, with an estimated threefold higher prevalence compared to women [5, 7]. The disease is also more predominant in white patients, who comprise 84% of affected individuals, and higher in high-income countries [8, 9]. Furthermore, studies have found increased prevalence of EoE in cold/arid climates along with urban settings [10, 11].

In addition to environmental factors, the disease pathogenesis is influenced by genetic susceptibility. Genome-wide association studies have identified over 40 specific genetic EoE-risk loci, several of which are associated with a variety of allergic conditions [12, 13]. Family studies have estimated the overall risk of developing

J. A. Klein
Department of Medicine, University of Chicago, Chicago, IL, USA
e-mail: Jeremy.Klein@uchicagomedicine.org

R. T. Kavitt (✉)
Center for Esophageal Diseases, Department of Medicine, Section of Gastroenterology, Hepatology, and Nutrition, University of Chicago, Chicago, IL, USA
e-mail: rkavitt@bsd.uchicago.edu

F. Schlottmann et al. (eds.), *Esophageal Disorders*,
https://doi.org/10.1007/978-3-032-08179-7_14

EoE to be 41% in monozygotic twins, 22% in dizygotic twins, and 2.4% in siblings, all higher than in the general population [14].

Diagnosis

Clinical Symptoms

The diagnosis of EoE relies on the combination of esophageal symptoms, endoscopic features, and at least 15 eosinophils per high-power field on histology. For infants and toddlers, maladaptive feeding behaviors are commonly present whereas vomiting, abdominal pain, and gastroesophageal reflux are more common later in childhood [15]. In contrast, dysphagia and food impactions are the most common presenting symptoms during the teenage years [16, 17]. For adults, the most common presenting symptom is dysphagia [18]. EoE is the culprit etiology in 12%–15% of patients presenting with dysphagia and ~50% in patients presenting with food impaction [18–20]. Esophageal inflammation with deposition of subepithelial fibrous tissue leads to remodeling and subsequent alterations in esophageal motility. These changes promote the progression of esophageal inflammation to fibrosis and stricture formation [21].

A prompt diagnosis is dependent on eliciting a comprehensive history of upper gastrointestinal symptoms and eating habits. It is important to note adaptive behaviors when obtaining a dysphagia history. These behaviors can include excessive fluids per bite, modifying foods to be smaller/easier to swallow, eating slowly, avoiding hard textures, and excessive chewing [22]. A detailed history of prior food impactions and therapeutic endoscopic dilations should be gathered. In addition, the close association with atopy including food allergies, asthma, and eczema should increase clinical suspicion for EoE [23].

In 2022, international experts created a consensus EoE severity scoring system called the "I-SEE" score that incorporates symptoms, endoscopy, and histology [24]. The "I-SEE" score can be useful for benchmarking EoE disease activity and tracking clinical response to therapeutics. Other useful clinical tools include the Dysphagia Symptom Questionnaire, Eosinophilic Esophagitis Activity Index patient-reported outcome score, and the Pediatric Eosinophilic Esophagitis Symptom Score [25–27].

Endoscopic Evaluation

The goals of endoscopy are to rule out alternative diagnoses, evaluate for distinctive endoscopic features, and obtain at least six biopsies from two esophageal levels for histologic analysis. Characteristic endoscopic findings include linear furrows, concentric rings, strictures, white exudates, and a decreased vascular pattern (edema). Linear furrows run longitudinally along the esophageal wall, whereas rings are located horizontally and are commonly referred to as trachealization [28]. The white exudate is composed of eosinophilic microabscesses, which can be confirmed on histology [29]. Studies have shown that exudates, furrows, and edema correlate with inflammation, whereas rings and stricturing reflect fibrotic remodeling [30, 31].

Additional esophageal abnormalities include feline esophagus (transient concentric rings that disappear with insufflation), narrow caliber esophagus, and crepe paper esophagus defined by mucosal fragility [32, 33]. Compared to adults, children with EoE tend to have a more normal-appearing esophagus, which could be attributed to less chronic inflammatory burden [34].

The updated 2025 ACG clinical guidelines suggest the routine use of the Eosinophilic Esophagitis Endoscopic Reference Score (EREFS) for patients with known EOE. EREFS includes separate scoring for each third of the esophagus and includes edema (0–2), rings (0–3), exudates (0–2), furrows (0–2), and strictures (0–1) [35]. The EREFS can be applied both at index endoscopy at time of diagnosis as well as subsequent endoscopies to monitor disease progression and trend response to therapy [36]. Follow-up studies note the EREFS score has only modest ability to predict histologic disease activity and response to treatment [37, 38].

Histologic Evaluation

Eosinophils are typically absent in the esophagus; thus, eosinophilic infiltration of the esophagus signifies pathology [39]. Several conditions can lead to eosinophil-mediated esophageal inflammation in addition to EoE. The etiology for secondary esophageal eosinophilia includes gastroesophageal reflux disease (GERD), eosinophilic gastrointestinal diseases (EGIDs), hypereosinophilic syndrome, celiac disease, Crohn's disease, achalasia, graft vs host disease, infection, drug hypersensitivity, among others [28]. EoE is a patchy condition and the preferred approach is to target areas of endoscopic inflammation and obtaining at least two to four biopsies from the proximal and distal esophagus (at least two distinct levels) [40].

The presence of 15 or more eosinophils in at least one microscopic high-power field (hpf) of both the proximal and distal esophageal epithelium is suggestive of an EoE diagnosis, but similar to clinical and endoscopic features, this alone cannot confirm EoE [31]. This threshold is applied to both adult and pediatric patients. Gastric and duodenal biopsies in asymptomatic patients are not routinely recommended [31].

Other Diagnostic Studies

To date, no noninvasive biomarkers exist to aid in EoE diagnosis, monitoring, or treatment. Several potential noninvasive biomarker (i.AQ1e. eosinophil cationic protein (ECP) and galectin-10 (CLC/GAL-10)) continue to be studied though none are currently cost-effective or recommended. Both serum immunoglobulin (Ig) E levels and peripheral eosinophilia are frequently elevated in EoE patients (along with allergic conditions and parasitic infections), but neither has adequate sensitivity and specificity to utilize in clinical practice [41, 42].

While EoE-related inflammation and fibrosis impacts esophageal function, esophageal manometry is not part of the diagnostic algorithm. There is no correlation between manometric motility findings with endoscopic features or symptoms [43]. A recent study of high-resolution manometry in EoE patients undergoing corticosteroid therapy also did not identify clear manometric parameters for treatment monitoring [44].

Other measurements of esophageal inflammation are being investigated, as endoscopy with esophageal biopsies is the current diagnostic standard of care. Furuta and colleagues reported that esophageal mucosal biopsies contain a high number of eosinophil granule proteins and developed a mechanism by which to obtain and measure these proteins using the Esophageal String Test (EnteroTrack) [45]. This study in children with EoE found that the quantity of the eosinophil-derived proteins correlated with mucosal inflammation [45]. A 2019 study found The String Test could distinguish active between inactive EoE (area under ROC of 0.83) [46]. Other researchers at the University of Cambridge examined the role of the Cytosponge as a minimally invasive way to collect esophageal tissue in EoE patients [47]. This study found the Cytosponge was well-tolerated, the number of collected eosinophils correlated with histology, and it offered high sensitivity and specificity (75% and 86%, respectively) [47, 48]. Further research is needed to expand knowledge of the efficacy of these methods before they are adapted as routine in clinical practice.

Impedance planimetry with Endoluminal Functional Lumen Imaging Probe (EndoFLIP, Crospon Medical Devices) has been utilized in EoE to evaluate esophageal mechanical properties [49]. In particular, EndoFLIP provides a more precise assessment of esophageal distensibility and can identify subtle strictures not seen endoscopically. However, given limited data and ongoing research, EndoFLIP is not routinely used in diagnostic or treatment decision making [50]. Radiographic studies are also not recommended to aid in diagnosing EoE, although barium radiography does have a limited utility in EoE patients for closer examination of esophageal strictures [51].

The Role of Proton Pump Inhibitors

The updated 2025 ACG guidelines no longer require a PPI trial prior to EoE diagnosis. Yet, PPIs still have an important role in initial EoE treatment. Along with antisecretory effects and improved esophageal barrier function, PPIs are anti-inflammatory and limit eosinophil trafficking to the esophagus by decreasing expression of eotaxin-3 [52, 53]. A 2024 retrospective cohort study of 305 newly diagnosed EoE patients found significantly higher rates of histologic remission with twice daily PPI compared to once daily dosing (54% vs. 12%, $p < .0001$) [54]. After an 8-week course, repeat endoscopy with biopsies is recommended to evaluate for persistent eosinophilic infiltration [55].

A large meta-analysis demonstrated symptomatic improvement after PPI use in 60% of patients with EoE and a histologic response in 50% [56]. No difference has been noted in PPI responsiveness between adult and pediatric patients. A 2015 study reported that around 27% of patients had histological relapse over a 1-year follow-up period and required subsequent PPI dose escalation [57]. Some patients eventually lose response to PPI therapy and require a change in mechanism to topical steroid or dupilumab.

All patients found to have 15 eosinophils per high-power field on biopsy who have not undergone a trial of proton pump inhibitor (PPI) therapy are recommended to initiate this treatment [58]. Given that GERD is the most common etiology of secondary esophageal eosinophilia, PPI treatment of GERD will likely result in improved GERD symptoms and a decreased number of eosinophils [59]. In the past, patients with a classic EoE presentation in whom GERD was excluded but had histologic response to PPI therapy were termed PPI-responsive esophageal eosinophilia (PPI-REE) [60]. At present time, PPI-REE is no longer recognized by the American College of Gastroenterology and the British Society of Gastroenterology.

Treatment

The treatment approach to EoE is categorized into elimination diets, medications, and dilation (Table 1). Selection of treatment depends on prior therapy and the severity of presentation, with the ultimate goals of improving symptoms and minimizing the risk of complications such as food impactions. Dietary therapy encompasses three possible approaches: the elemental diet, the allergy test–directed elimination diet, and the empiric elimination diet (6- and 4-food subtypes). Pharmacologic therapy ranges from PPIs and topical corticosteroids to the monoclonal antibody dupilumab and emerging biologics that target IL-13 (Cendakimab), IL-5 (Benralizumab), or the siglec-8 receptor (lirentelimab). Patients with symptomatic fibrostenotic disease or refractory symptoms may benefit from endoscopic dilation (in addition to anti-inflammatory therapy).

Dietary Therapy

Dietary allergens are associated with EoE in both pediatric and adult populations and carefully designed dietary modifications offer a nonpharmacologic treatment option [61]. The diet strategy is influenced by patient preference and should ideally involve both an allergist and a dietician to maximize efficacy and practicality. Dietitian support (including a feeding therapist if available) is important for all EoE dietary therapies to increase adherence and minimize the risk of inadequate nutrition intake (particularly with pediatric patients).

Elemental Diet

The elemental diet is the strictest dietary plan and also the most effective, inducing histologic remission in 90.8% of patients [62]. The diet is free of allergens and

Table 1 Eosinophilic esophagitis treatment summary

Therapy	Description/findings
Dietary therapy	
Elemental diet	Amino acid–based, allergen-free formula followed by slow reintroduction of foods Most effective but also most strict, causing difficulty with adherence
Allergy testing–directed elimination diet	Elimination of food groups based on allergy testing Overall poor efficacy and the least favored of the three dietary regimens
Empiric elimination diet	Six most commonly allergenic food groups (milk, soy, egg, wheat, peanut/tree nuts, shellfish/fish) are removed from the diet and slowly, individually reintroduced after a symptomatic and histologic response
Pharmacologic therapy	
Proton pump inhibitors	Used as initial therapy for EoE Omeprazole 40 mg daily or other equivalent PPI
Topical corticosteroids	Used for initial and maintenance therapy in eosinophilic esophagitis unresponsive to proton pump inhibitor therapy Budesonide viscous suspension 1–2 mg/day for children or 2–4 mg/day for adults, typically in a divided dose, or fluticasone via metered-dose inhaler 110–880 μg/day in a divided dose for children or 1760 μg/day in a divided dose for adults
Dupilumab	Used as "step-up" therapy for refractory symptoms on PPI or other therapy 300 mg subcutaneously every week (if ≥40 kg), 300 mg every other week (if 30 to <40 kg), and 200 mg every other week (if 15 to <30 kg).
Endoscopic treatment	
Endoscopic dilation	Usually reserved for patients who relapse on dietary or pharmacologic therapy First-line therapy if high-grade strictures are present

The dosing listed in the table is based on the 2025 American College of Gastroenterology guidelines

based on a formula of amino acids, basic carbohydrates, and medium-chain triglycerides [63]. The majority of studies evaluating the elemental diet have been conducted in the pediatric population, demonstrating its effectiveness in improving both symptoms and histologic inflammation [34, 64, 65]. Studies in adults also demonstrate efficacy and remission [62, 66]. The main limitation of the elemental diet is the very narrow profile which limits long-term adherence. After achieving clinical and histologic remissions, foods can be reintroduced under close monitoring. The diet is frequently reserved for those who lack response to other therapies, and practitioners may need to use enteral feeding modalities to reach nutritional needs [67].

Allergy Testing–Directed Elimination Diet

Food allergy testing guides therapy in the allergy testing–directed elimination diet. Patients undergo skin-prick testing or radioallergosorbent testing to identify specific allergens [30]. Large variability has been reported in the effectiveness of this dietary approach. A study in the pediatric population demonstrated histologic remission in 77% of patients, whereas a study in adults showed a poorer response of 34% [68,

69]. A meta-analysis of both children and adults concluded that only 45.5% of patients achieved histologic remission [62]. Overall, this dietary approach is limited by a poor demonstrated association between allergens identified by the standard testing protocols and EoE exacerbation [70, 71]. Current guidelines recommend against testing for allergens as they are not well correlated with predicting EoE triggers [72].

Empiric Elimination Diet

The empiric elimination diet is the least restrictive of the three methods and the most extensively studied. In the 6-food elimination diet, the nutrition plan is altered by removing six potential allergens: milk, wheat, egg, soy, nuts, and seafood [73]. After confirmed symptomatic and histologic improvements, the food groups are slowly and individually reintroduced with most patients isolating one or two food triggers. After reintroduction, the most commonly identified food trigger is wheat (60%) and dairy (50%) [74]. Histologic remission has occurred in 72%–73% of patients using this therapy [62, 75]. As compared to 6-food, the alternative 4-food elimination diet withholds dairy, wheat, egg. It is less studied (and less efficacious compared to 6-food), but provides an alternative for patients wishing to decrease the amount of dietary restrictions [67]. One study found 54% of patients achieved clinicopathologic response [76]. A 2023 multicenter randomized control trial found 1-food elimination diets achieved similar remission rates and comparable histologic/endoscopic improvement as compared to 6-food elimination diets [77]. This trial promotes eliminating animal milk alone as an efficacious and practical diet for EoE.

Pharmacologic Therapy

Pharmacologic therapy includes PPIs, topical corticosteroids, systemic corticosteroids, monoclonal antibodies and biologics. In September of 2022, the United States Food and Drug Administration (FDA) approved dupilumab as the first treatment for EoE. Dupilumab is a monoclonal antibody against the interleukin-4 receptor alpha (IL-4rα) that targets the type-2 inflammatory cascade by blocking the effect of both IL-4 and IL-13. Several other antibody-directed agents are currently being studied and will not be described further in this article.

Topical Corticosteroids

Topical corticosteroids are often used as first-line agents once an EoE diagnosis is confirmed [31, 78]. Corticosteroids decrease eosinophil mucosal migration by inhibiting cytokines, leading to reduced remodeling and tissue fibrosis [79, 80]. This regimen offers a favorable safety profile; the most commonly cited side effect is candidiasis, and compared to systemic corticosteroids, adrenal axis suppression is rare [81].

Both fluticasone administered via a metered-dose inhaler and viscous budesonide swallowed in a liquid slurry have shown efficacy when initiated with an 8-week twice-daily trial [50, 55, 82]. Budesonide oral suspension (BOS) was approved by the US FDA in February 2024 for patients age 11 years or older. At the time of publication, the fluticasone propionate orally disintegrating tablet remains under investigation in phase 3 clinical trials. Studies comparing fluticasone to placebo in both adults and children reported a 50%–65% remission rate [83, 84]. Randomized controlled trials of budesonide vs placebo also highlight significant improvement in symptoms and eosinophil burden on histology [85, 86]. A 2019 randomized, double-blind clinical trial compared budesonide slurry to swallowed meter dosed inhaler fluticasone in PPI non-responsive patients with EoE. The study found similar rates of histologic response (71% in budesonide vs. 64% in fluticasone) along with similar dysphagia and EREF scores [87]. Updated ACG guidelines from 2025 recommend either fluticasone MDI or budesonide slurry for initial treatment.

Systemic Corticosteroids

Limited data exist regarding the use of systemic corticosteroids in EoE. A randomized, controlled trial comparing oral prednisone to topical fluticasone demonstrated no significant difference in clinical and histologic improvements [88]. However, 40% of patients who received prednisone experienced systemic adverse effects compared to no systemic effects in the fluticasone group [88]. In practice, systemic corticosteroids are not recommended by the current guidelines and are reserved for severe refractory cases or instances in which a rapid response is needed.

Dupilumab

Dupilumab is a monoclonal antibody that targets the interluekon-4 receptor alpha (IL-4rα) to block the cytokine cascade responsible for EoE-related inflammation [89]. It was first approved by the FDA in March of 2017 for adults with moderate-to-severe atopic dermatitis. As mentioned above, dupilumab was then FDA approved in September of 2022 for EoE and expanded to ages 1 through 11 in February of 2024.

The pivotal randomized control trial (RCT) published in December 2022 found that 60% of patients achieved histologic remission at 24 weeks with subcutaneous dupilumab (300 mg, dosed every 7 days) compared to 5% treated with placebo ($p < .0001$). When assessing for symptomatic relief according to the Dysphagia Symptom Questionnaire, the weekly dosing was more effective than every other week (21.9 point decrease vs. 9.6 points; $p < .001$) [90]. Notably, the RCT was compromised of a medically refractory cohort; all patients were PPI nonresponsive, 40% with prior esophageal dilation, and 50% with no response to topical steroids or intolerance [50].

For patients who remain symptomatic after a trial of topical corticosteroids, dupilumab can be utilized for step-up therapy in most cases. In general, dupilumab is very well tolerated with the most common side effects being injections site reaction, upper respiratory infections, mild conjunctivitis, and a small risk for arthralgia. There is no immunogenicity concerns at present time and screening for Tuberculosis or hepatitis prior to therapy initiation is not required.

Endoscopic Dilation Therapy

Endoscopic treatment is recommended for patients with a high-grade stricture or those who clinically relapse despite dietary or pharmacologic therapy. Dilation does not have an effect on eosinophilic infiltration or underlying inflammation [91]. Therefore, updated clinical guidance recommends pairing dilation with anti-inflammatory agents as this can prevent serial dilations after histologic response is observed [92]. The technique can be performed using either a bougie dilator or a through-the-scope balloon. No data exist demonstrating the superiority of one technique over another [55]. A conservative gradual approach to dilation is recommended to avoid complications, with the objective to dilate the esophagus between 15 and 18 mm in diameter [93]. Success of endoscopic dilation, defined by symptom improvement, occurs in 75%–83% of patients [94, 95]. However, dilation may not clinically benefit patients without severe strictures [96]. Serial dilations are often performed to attain symptom response. A study of 164 EoE patients who underwent dilation concluded that 75% required repeat dilation within 1 year [97].

Esophageal perforation is rarely seen in EoE and can result from food impaction, prolonged retching, or mechanical dilation [98, 99]. A retrospective examination of 511 patients estimated the risk of perforation in EoE at 2%, with 80% of cases resulting from a prolonged food impaction [97]. Studies investigating the risk of perforation after dilation therapy found the perforation rate to be below 1% [94, 99, 100].

Summary

EoE is a chronic and relapsing inflammatory condition. It is one of the leading causes of dysphagia and food impactions. Diagnosis requires the presence of esophageal symptoms along with esophageal eosinophilia confirmed on histologic analysis. There is currently no longer a role for PPI responsiveness in the diagnostic pathway of EoE. Instead, PPI use is viewed as part of the treatment algorithm for newly diagnosed EoE. Existing treatment strategies target the underlying inflammation and aim to provide symptomatic relief (based on Dysphasia Symptom Questionnaire) along with endoscopic and histologic improvement. Patients with confirmed EoE are initiated on twice daily PPI, topical corticosteroids, or empiric elimination diets. For those patients with persistent symptoms or evidence of ongoing inflammation or strictures, therapy can be stepped-up to dupilumab. In the presence of unrelenting symptoms on therapy or severe stricturing disease, repeat endoscopy with dilation can be performed. Multiple biologics including monoclonal antibodies and additional corticosteroid formulations are undergoing further investigation and could be available soon. The goals of EoE treatment are to improve symptoms and quality of life by decreasing esophageal eosinophilic infiltration and preventing disease progression.

References

1. Landres RT, Kuster GG, Strum WB. Eosinophilic esophagitis in a patient with vigorous achalasia. Gastroenterology. 1978;74(6):1298–301.
2. Dellon ES. Epidemiology of eosinophilic esophagitis. Gastroenterol Clin N Am. 2014;43(2):201–18. https://doi.org/10.1016/j.gtc.2014.02.002.
3. Hahn JW, Lee K, Shin JI, et al. Global incidence and prevalence of eosinophilic esophagitis, 1976-2022: a systematic review and meta-analysis. Clin Gastroenterol Hepatol. 2023;21(13):3270–3284.e77. https://doi.org/10.1016/j.cgh.2023.06.005.
4. Croese J, Fairley SK, Masson JW, et al. Clinical and endoscopic features of eosinophilic esophagitis in adults. Gastrointest Endosc. 2003;58(4):516–22.
5. Kapel RC, Miller JK, Torres C, Aksoy S, Lash R, Katzka DA. Eosinophilic esophagitis: a prevalent disease in the United States that affects all age groups. Gastroenterology. 2008;134(5):1316–21. https://doi.org/10.1053/j.gastro.2008.02.016.
6. Dellon ES, Jensen ET, Martin CF, Shaheen NJ, Kappelman MD. Prevalence of eosinophilic esophagitis in the United States. Clin Gastroenterol Hepatol. 2014;12(4):589–96.e1. https://doi.org/10.1016/j.cgh.2013.09.008.
7. Arias A, Perez-Martinez I, Tenias JM, Lucendo AJ. Systematic review with meta-analysis: the incidence and prevalence of eosinophilic oesophagitis in children and adults in population-based studies. Aliment Pharmacol Ther. 2016;43(1):3–15. https://doi.org/10.1111/apt.13441.
8. Franciosi JP, Tam V, Liacouras CA, Spergel JM. A case-control study of sociodemographic and geographic characteristics of 335 children with eosinophilic esophagitis. Clin Gastroenterol Hepatol. 2009;7(4):415–9. https://doi.org/10.1016/j.cgh.2008.10.006.
9. Sperry SL, Woosley JT, Shaheen NJ, Dellon ES. Influence of race and gender on the presentation of eosinophilic esophagitis. Am J Gastroenterol. 2012;107(2):215–21. https://doi.org/10.1038/ajg.2011.342.
10. Hurrell JM, Genta RM, Dellon ES. Prevalence of esophageal eosinophilia varies by climate zone in the United States. Am J Gastroenterol. 2012;107(5):698–706. https://doi.org/10.1038/ajg.2012.6.
11. Spergel JM, Book WM, Mays E, et al. Variation in prevalence, diagnostic criteria, and initial management options for eosinophilic gastrointestinal diseases in the United States. J Pediatr Gastroenterol Nutr. 2011;52(3):300–6. https://doi.org/10.1097/MPG.0b013e3181eb5a9f.
12. Kottyan LC, Rothenberg ME. Genetics of eosinophilic esophagitis. Mucosal Immunol. 2017;10(3):580–8. https://doi.org/10.1038/mi.2017.4.
13. Kottyan LC, Parameswaran S, Weirauch MT, Rothenberg ME, Martin LJ. The genetic etiology of eosinophilic esophagitis. J Allergy Clin Immunol. 2020;145(1):9–15. https://doi.org/10.1016/j.jaci.2019.11.013.
14. Alexander ES, Martin LJ, Collins MH, et al. Twin and family studies reveal strong environmental and weaker genetic cues explaining heritability of eosinophilic esophagitis. J Allergy Clin Immunol. 2014;134(5):1084–1092.e1. https://doi.org/10.1016/j.jaci.2014.07.021.
15. Mukkada VA, Haas A, Maune NC, et al. Feeding dysfunction in children with eosinophilic gastrointestinal diseases. Pediatrics. 2010;126(3):e672–7. https://doi.org/10.1542/peds.2009-2227.
16. Noel RJ, Putnam PE, Rothenberg ME. Eosinophilic esophagitis. N Engl J Med. 2004;351(9):940–1. https://doi.org/10.1056/NEJM200408263510924.
17. Assa'ad AH, Putnam PE, Collins MH, et al. Pediatric patients with eosinophilic esophagitis: an 8-year follow-up. J Allergy Clin Immunol. 2007;119(3):731–8. https://doi.org/10.1016/j.jaci.2006.10.044.
18. Prasad GA, Talley NJ, Romero Y, et al. Prevalence and predictive factors of eosinophilic esophagitis in patients presenting with dysphagia: a prospective study. Am J Gastroenterol. 2007;102(12):2627–32. https://doi.org/10.1111/j.1572-0241.2007.01512.x.

19. Kerlin P, Jones D, Remedios M, Campbell C. Prevalence of eosinophilic esophagitis in adults with food bolus obstruction of the esophagus. J Clin Gastroenterol. 2007;41(4):356–61. https://doi.org/10.1097/01.mcg.0000225590.08825.77.
20. Sperry SL, Crockett SD, Miller CB, Shaheen NJ, Dellon ES. Esophageal foreign-body impactions: epidemiology, time trends, and the impact of the increasing prevalence of eosinophilic esophagitis. Gastrointest Endosc. 2011;74(5):985–91. https://doi.org/10.1016/j.gie.2011.06.029.
21. Dellon ES, Kim HP, Sperry SL, Rybnicek DA, Woosley JT, Shaheen NJ. A phenotypic analysis shows that eosinophilic esophagitis is a progressive fibrostenotic disease. Gastrointest Endosc. 2014;79(4):577–85.e4. https://doi.org/10.1016/j.gie.2013.10.027.
22. Hirano I, Furuta GT. Approaches and challenges to management of pediatric and adult patients with eosinophilic esophagitis. Gastroenterology. 2020;158(4):840–51. https://doi.org/10.1053/j.gastro.2019.09.052.
23. Lucendo AJ, Sanchez-Cazalilla M. Adult versus pediatric eosinophilic esophagitis: important differences and similarities for the clinician to understand. Expert Rev Clin Immunol. 2012;8(8):733–45. https://doi.org/10.1586/eci.12.68.
24. Dellon ES, Khoury P, Muir AB, et al. A clinical severity index for eosinophilic esophagitis: development, consensus, and future directions. Gastroenterology. 2022;163(1):59–76. https://doi.org/10.1053/j.gastro.2022.03.025.
25. Schoepfer AM, Straumann A, Panczak R, et al. Development and validation of a symptom-based activity index for adults with eosinophilic esophagitis. Gastroenterology. 2014;147(6):1255–66.e21. https://doi.org/10.1053/j.gastro.2014.08.028.
26. Martin LJ, Franciosi JP, Collins MH, et al. Pediatric Eosinophilic Esophagitis Symptom Scores (PEESS v2.0) identify histologic and molecular correlates of the key clinical features of disease. J Allergy Clin Immunol. 2015;135(6):1519–28.e8. https://doi.org/10.1016/j.jaci.2015.03.004.
27. Dellon ES, Irani AM, Hill MR, Hirano I. Development and field testing of a novel patient-reported outcome measure of dysphagia in patients with eosinophilic esophagitis. Aliment Pharmacol Ther. 2013;38(6):634–42. https://doi.org/10.1111/apt.12413.
28. Abe Y, Sasaki Y, Yagi M, Yaoita T, Nishise S, Ueno Y. Diagnosis and treatment of eosinophilic esophagitis in clinical practice. Clin J Gastroenterol. 2017;10(2):87–102. https://doi.org/10.1007/s12328-017-0725-4.
29. Lim JR, Gupta SK, Croffie JM, et al. White specks in the esophageal mucosa: an endoscopic manifestation of non-reflux eosinophilic esophagitis in children. Gastrointest Endosc. 2004;59(7):835–8.
30. Furuta GT, Liacouras CA, Collins MH, et al. Eosinophilic esophagitis in children and adults: a systematic review and consensus recommendations for diagnosis and treatment. Gastroenterology. 2007;133(4):1342–63. https://doi.org/10.1053/j.gastro.2007.08.017.
31. Liacouras CA, Furuta GT, Hirano I, et al. Eosinophilic esophagitis: updated consensus recommendations for children and adults. J Allergy Clin Immunol. 2011;128(1):3–20.e6; quiz 21–2. https://doi.org/10.1016/j.jaci.2011.02.040.
32. Kaplan M, Mutlu EA, Jakate S, et al. Endoscopy in eosinophilic esophagitis: "feline" esophagus and perforation risk. Clin Gastroenterol Hepatol. 2003;1(6):433–7.
33. Straumann A, Spichtin HP, Grize L, Bucher KA, Beglinger C, Simon HU. Natural history of primary eosinophilic esophagitis: a follow-up of 30 adult patients for up to 11.5 years. Gastroenterology. 2003;125(6):1660–9.
34. Liacouras CA, Spergel JM, Ruchelli E, et al. Eosinophilic esophagitis: a 10-year experience in 381 children. Clin Gastroenterol Hepatol. 2005;3(12):1198–206.
35. Hirano I, Moy N, Heckman MG, Thomas CS, Gonsalves N, Achem SR. Endoscopic assessment of the oesophageal features of eosinophilic oesophagitis: validation of a novel classification and grading system. Gut. 2013;62(4):489–95. https://doi.org/10.1136/gutjnl-2011-301817.

36. Dellon ES, Cotton CC, Gebhart JH, et al. Accuracy of the eosinophilic esophagitis endoscopic reference score in diagnosis and determining response to treatment. Clin Gastroenterol Hepatol. 2016;14(1):31–9. https://doi.org/10.1016/j.cgh.2015.08.040.
37. van Rhijn BD, Verheij J, Smout AJ, Bredenoord AJ. The endoscopic reference score shows modest accuracy to predict histologic remission in adult patients with eosinophilic esophagitis. Neurogastroenterol Motil. 2016;28(11):1714–22. https://doi.org/10.1111/nmo.12872.
38. Rodriguez-Sanchez J, Barrio-Andres J, Nantes Castillejo O, et al. The endoscopic reference score shows modest accuracy to predict either clinical or histological activity in adult patients with eosinophilic oesophagitis. Aliment Pharmacol Ther. 2017;45(2):300–9. https://doi.org/10.1111/apt.13845.
39. Matsushita T, Maruyama R, Ishikawa N, et al. The number and distribution of eosinophils in the adult human gastrointestinal tract: a study and comparison of racial and environmental factors. Am J Surg Pathol. 2015;39(4):521–7. https://doi.org/10.1097/PAS.0000000000000370.
40. Aceves SS, Alexander JA, Baron TH, et al. Endoscopic approach to eosinophilic esophagitis: American Society for Gastrointestinal Endoscopy consensus conference. Gastrointest Endosc. 2022;96(4):576–592.e1. https://doi.org/10.1016/j.gie.2022.05.013.
41. Erwin EA, James HR, Gutekunst HM, Russo JM, Kelleher KJ, Platts-Mills TA. Serum IgE measurement and detection of food allergy in pediatric patients with eosinophilic esophagitis. Ann Allergy Asthma Immunol. 2010;104(6):496–502. https://doi.org/10.1016/j.anai.2010.03.018.
42. Dellon ES, Gibbs WB, Fritchie KJ, et al. Clinical, endoscopic, and histologic findings distinguish eosinophilic esophagitis from gastroesophageal reflux disease. Clin Gastroenterol Hepatol. 2009;7(12):1305–13; quiz 1261. https://doi.org/10.1016/j.cgh.2009.08.030.
43. von Arnim U, Kandulski A, Weigt J, Malfertheiner P. Correlation of high-resolution manometric findings with symptoms of dysphagia and endoscopic features in adults with eosinophilic esophagitis. Dig Dis. 2017;35:472–7. https://doi.org/10.1159/000458407.
44. Nennstiel S, Bajbouj M, Becker V, et al. High-resolution manometry in patients with eosinophilic esophagitis under topical steroid therapy-a prospective observational study (HIMEOS-study). Neurogastroenterol Motil. 2016;28(4):599–607. https://doi.org/10.1111/nmo.12753.
45. Furuta GT, Kagalwalla AF, Lee JJ, et al. The oesophageal string test: a novel, minimally invasive method measures mucosal inflammation in eosinophilic oesophagitis. Gut. 2013;62(10):1395–405. https://doi.org/10.1136/gutjnl-2012-303171.
46. Ackerman SJ, Kagalwalla AF, Hirano I, et al. One-hour esophageal string test: a nonendoscopic minimally invasive test that accurately detects disease activity in eosinophilic esophagitis. Am J Gastroenterol. 2019;114(10):1614–25. https://doi.org/10.14309/ajg.0000000000000371.
47. Katzka DA, Geno DM, Ravi A, et al. Accuracy, safety, and tolerability of tissue collection by Cytosponge vs endoscopy for evaluation of eosinophilic esophagitis. Clin Gastroenterol Hepatol. 2015;13(1):77–83.e2. https://doi.org/10.1016/j.cgh.2014.06.026.
48. Katzka DA, Smyrk TC, Alexander JA, et al. Accuracy and safety of the Cytosponge for assessing histologic activity in eosinophilic esophagitis: a two-center study. Am J Gastroenterol. 2017;112(10):1538–44. https://doi.org/10.1038/ajg.2017.244.
49. Kwiatek MA, Hirano I, Kahrilas PJ, Rothe J, Luger D, Pandolfino JE. Mechanical properties of the esophagus in eosinophilic esophagitis. Gastroenterology. 2011;140(1):82–90. https://doi.org/10.1053/j.gastro.2010.09.037.
50. Dellon ES, Muir AB, Katzka DA, et al. ACG clinical guideline: diagnosis and management of eosinophilic esophagitis. Am J Gastroenterol. 2025;120(1):31–59. https://doi.org/10.14309/ajg.0000000000003194.
51. Binkovitz LA, Lorenz EA, Di Lorenzo C, Kahwash S. Pediatric eosinophilic esophagitis: radiologic findings with pathologic correlation. Pediatr Radiol. 2010;40(5):714–9. https://doi.org/10.1007/s00247-009-1484-2.
52. Cheng E, Zhang X, Huo X, et al. Omeprazole blocks eotaxin-3 expression by oesophageal squamous cells from patients with eosinophilic oesophagitis and GORD. Gut. 2013;62(6):824–32. https://doi.org/10.1136/gutjnl-2012-302250.

53. van Rhijn BD, Weijenborg PW, Verheij J, et al. Proton pump inhibitors partially restore mucosal integrity in patients with proton pump inhibitor-responsive esophageal eosinophilia but not eosinophilic esophagitis. Clin Gastroenterol Hepatol. 2014;12(11):1815–23.e2. https://doi.org/10.1016/j.cgh.2014.02.037.
54. Muftah M, Goldin AH, Barshop K, et al. Twice-daily proton pump inhibitor induces higher remission rate in eosinophilic esophagitis than once-daily regimen regardless of total daily dose. Am J Gastroenterol. 2024;119(5):991–5. https://doi.org/10.14309/ajg.0000000000002712.
55. Dellon ES, Gonsalves N, Hirano I, et al. ACG clinical guideline: evidenced based approach to the diagnosis and management of esophageal eosinophilia and eosinophilic esophagitis (EoE). Am J Gastroenterol. 2013;108(5):679–92; quiz 693. https://doi.org/10.1038/ajg.2013.71.
56. Lucendo AJ, Arias A, Molina-Infante J. Efficacy of proton pump inhibitor drugs for inducing clinical and histologic remission in patients with symptomatic esophageal eosinophilia: a systematic review and meta-analysis. Clin Gastroenterol Hepatol. 2016;14(1):13–22.e1. https://doi.org/10.1016/j.cgh.2015.07.041.
57. Molina-Infante J, Rodriguez-Sanchez J, Martinek J, et al. Long-term loss of response in proton pump inhibitor-responsive esophageal eosinophilia is uncommon and influenced by CYP2C19 genotype and rhinoconjunctivitis. Am J Gastroenterol. 2015;110(11):1567–75. https://doi.org/10.1038/ajg.2015.314.
58. Dellon ES. Diagnostics of eosinophilic esophagitis: clinical, endoscopic, and histologic pitfalls. Dig Dis. 2014;32(1–2):48–53. https://doi.org/10.1159/000357009.
59. Rothenberg ME. Biology and treatment of eosinophilic esophagitis. Gastroenterology. 2009;137(4):1238–49. https://doi.org/10.1053/j.gastro.2009.07.007.
60. Straumann A, Schoepfer A. Update on basic and clinical aspects of eosinophilic oesophagitis. Gut. 2014;63(8):1355–63. https://doi.org/10.1136/gutjnl-2013-306414.
61. Redd M, Schey R. Eosinophilic esophagitis: current treatment. Dig Dis Sci. 2013;58(3):613–20. https://doi.org/10.1007/s10620-012-2383-1.
62. Arias A, Gonzalez-Cervera J, Tenias JM, Lucendo AJ. Efficacy of dietary interventions for inducing histologic remission in patients with eosinophilic esophagitis: a systematic review and meta-analysis. Gastroenterology. 2014;146(7):1639–48. https://doi.org/10.1053/j.gastro.2014.02.006.
63. Dellon ES. Diagnosis and management of eosinophilic esophagitis. Clin Gastroenterol Hepatol. 2012;10(10):1066–78. https://doi.org/10.1016/j.cgh.2012.06.003.
64. Markowitz JE, Spergel JM, Ruchelli E, Liacouras CA. Elemental diet is an effective treatment for eosinophilic esophagitis in children and adolescents. Am J Gastroenterol. 2003;98(4):777–82. https://doi.org/10.1111/j.1572-0241.2003.07390.x.
65. Henderson CJ, Abonia JP, King EC, et al. Comparative dietary therapy effectiveness in remission of pediatric eosinophilic esophagitis. J Allergy Clin Immunol. 2012;129(6):1570–8. https://doi.org/10.1016/j.jaci.2012.03.023.
66. Peterson KA, Byrne KR, Vinson LA, et al. Elemental diet induces histologic response in adult eosinophilic esophagitis. Am J Gastroenterol. 2013;108(5):759–66. https://doi.org/10.1038/ajg.2012.468.
67. Groetch M, Venter C, Skypala I, et al. Dietary therapy and nutrition management of eosinophilic esophagitis: a work group report of the American Academy of Allergy, Asthma, and Immunology. J Allergy Clin Immunol Pract. 2017;5(2):312–324.e29. https://doi.org/10.1016/j.jaip.2016.12.026.
68. Spergel JM, Brown-Whitehorn TF, Cianferoni A, et al. Identification of causative foods in children with eosinophilic esophagitis treated with an elimination diet. J Allergy Clin Immunol. 2012;130(2):461–7.e5. https://doi.org/10.1016/j.jaci.2012.05.021.
69. Molina-Infante J, Martin-Noguerol E, Alvarado-Arenas M, Porcel-Carreno SL, Jimenez-Timon S, Hernandez-Arbeiza FJ. Selective elimination diet based on skin testing has suboptimal efficacy for adult eosinophilic esophagitis. J Allergy Clin Immunol. 2012;130(5):1200–2. https://doi.org/10.1016/j.jaci.2012.06.027.

70. Sampson HA, Aceves S, Bock SA, et al. Food allergy: a practice parameter update-2014. J Allergy Clin Immunol. 2014;134(5):1016–25.e43. https://doi.org/10.1016/j.jaci.2014.05.013.
71. van Rhijn BD, Vlieg-Boerstra BJ, Versteeg SA, et al. Evaluation of allergen-microarray-guided dietary intervention as treatment of eosinophilic esophagitis. J Allergy Clin Immunol. 2015;136(4):1095–7.e3. https://doi.org/10.1016/j.jaci.2015.02.038.
72. Spergel JM, Andrews T, Brown-Whitehorn TF, Beausoleil JL, Liacouras CA. Treatment of eosinophilic esophagitis with specific food elimination diet directed by a combination of skin prick and patch tests. Ann Allergy Asthma Immunol. 2005;95(4):336–43. https://doi.org/10.1016/S1081-1206(10)61151-9.
73. Kagalwalla AF, Sentongo TA, Ritz S, et al. Effect of six-food elimination diet on clinical and histologic outcomes in eosinophilic esophagitis. Clin Gastroenterol Hepatol. 2006;4(9):1097–102. https://doi.org/10.1016/j.cgh.2006.05.026.
74. Gonsalves N, Yang GY, Doerfler B, Ritz S, Ditto AM, Hirano I. Elimination diet effectively treats eosinophilic esophagitis in adults; food reintroduction identifies causative factors. Gastroenterology. 2012;142(7):1451–9.e1; quiz e14–5. https://doi.org/10.1053/j.gastro.2012.03.001.
75. Lucendo AJ, Arias A, Gonzalez-Cervera J, et al. Empiric 6-food elimination diet induced and maintained prolonged remission in patients with adult eosinophilic esophagitis: a prospective study on the food cause of the disease. J Allergy Clin Immunol. 2013;131(3):797–804. https://doi.org/10.1016/j.jaci.2012.12.664.
76. Molina-Infante J, Arias A, Barrio J, Rodriguez-Sanchez J, Sanchez-Cazalilla M, Lucendo AJ. Four-food group elimination diet for adult eosinophilic esophagitis: a prospective multicenter study. J Allergy Clin Immunol. 2014;134(5):1093–9.e1. https://doi.org/10.1016/j.jaci.2014.07.023.
77. Kliewer KL, Gonsalves N, Dellon ES, et al. One-food versus six-food elimination diet therapy for the treatment of eosinophilic oesophagitis: a multicentre, randomised, open-label trial. Lancet Gastroenterol Hepatol. 2023;8(5):408–21. https://doi.org/10.1016/S2468-1253(23)00012-2.
78. Chuang MY, Chinnaratha MA, Hancock DG, et al. Topical steroid therapy for the treatment of eosinophilic esophagitis (EoE): a systematic review and meta-analysis. Clin Transl Gastroenterol. 2015;6:e82. https://doi.org/10.1038/ctg.2015.9.
79. Aceves SS, Newbury RO, Chen D, et al. Resolution of remodeling in eosinophilic esophagitis correlates with epithelial response to topical corticosteroids. Allergy. 2010;65(1):109–16. https://doi.org/10.1111/j.1398-9995.2009.02142.x.
80. Kagalwalla AF, Akhtar N, Woodruff SA, et al. Eosinophilic esophagitis: epithelial mesenchymal transition contributes to esophageal remodeling and reverses with treatment. J Allergy Clin Immunol. 2012;129(5):1387–1396.e7. https://doi.org/10.1016/j.jaci.2012.03.005.
81. Furuta GT, Katzka DA. Eosinophilic esophagitis. N Engl J Med. 2015;373(17):1640–8. https://doi.org/10.1056/NEJMra1502863.
82. Albert D, Heifert TA, Min SB, et al. Comparisons of fluticasone to budesonide in the treatment of eosinophilic esophagitis. Dig Dis Sci. 2016;61(7):1996–2001. https://doi.org/10.1007/s10620-016-4110-9.
83. Konikoff MR, Noel RJ, Blanchard C, et al. A randomized, double-blind, placebo-controlled trial of fluticasone propionate for pediatric eosinophilic esophagitis. Gastroenterology. 2006;131(5):1381–91. https://doi.org/10.1053/j.gastro.2006.08.033.
84. Butz BK, Wen T, Gleich GJ, et al. Efficacy, dose reduction, and resistance to high-dose fluticasone in patients with eosinophilic esophagitis. Gastroenterology. 2014;147(2):324–33.e5. https://doi.org/10.1053/j.gastro.2014.04.019.
85. Dohil R, Newbury R, Fox L, Bastian J, Aceves S. Oral viscous budesonide is effective in children with eosinophilic esophagitis in a randomized, placebo-controlled trial. Gastroenterology. 2010;139(2):418–29. https://doi.org/10.1053/j.gastro.2010.05.001.
86. Straumann A, Conus S, Degen L, et al. Long-term budesonide maintenance treatment is partially effective for patients with eosinophilic esophagitis. Clin Gastroenterol Hepatol. 2011;9(5):400–9.e1. https://doi.org/10.1016/j.cgh.2011.01.017.

87. Dellon ES, Woosley JT, Arrington A, et al. Efficacy of budesonide vs fluticasone for initial treatment of eosinophilic esophagitis in a randomized controlled trial. Gastroenterology. 2019;157(1):65–73.e5. https://doi.org/10.1053/j.gastro.2019.03.014.
88. Schaefer ET, Fitzgerald JF, Molleston JP, et al. Comparison of oral prednisone and topical fluticasone in the treatment of eosinophilic esophagitis: a randomized trial in children. Clin Gastroenterol Hepatol. 2008;6(2):165–73. https://doi.org/10.1016/j.cgh.2007.11.008.
89. Gandhi NA, Pirozzi G, Graham NMH. Commonality of the IL-4/IL-13 pathway in atopic diseases. Expert Rev Clin Immunol. 2017;13(5):425–37. https://doi.org/10.1080/1744666X.2017.1298443.
90. Dellon ES, Rothenberg ME, Collins MH, et al. Dupilumab in adults and adolescents with eosinophilic esophagitis. N Engl J Med. 2022;387(25):2317–30. https://doi.org/10.1056/NEJMoa2205982.
91. Singla MB, Moawad FJ. An overview of the diagnosis and management of eosinophilic esophagitis. Clin Transl Gastroenterol. 2016;7:e155. https://doi.org/10.1038/ctg.2016.4.
92. Schupack DA, Ravi K, Geno DM, et al. Effect of maintenance therapy for eosinophilic esophagitis on need for recurrent dilation. Dig Dis Sci. 2021;66(2):503–10. https://doi.org/10.1007/s10620-020-06192-8.
93. Richter JE. Esophageal dilation in eosinophilic esophagitis. Best Pract Res Clin Gastroenterol. 2015;29(5):815–28. https://doi.org/10.1016/j.bpg.2015.06.015.
94. Moawad FJ, Cheatham JG, DeZee KJ. Meta-analysis: the safety and efficacy of dilation in eosinophilic oesophagitis. Aliment Pharmacol Ther. 2013;38(7):713–20. https://doi.org/10.1111/apt.12438.
95. Dellon ES, Gibbs WB, Rubinas TC, et al. Esophageal dilation in eosinophilic esophagitis: safety and predictors of clinical response and complications. Gastrointest Endosc. 2010;71(4):706–12. https://doi.org/10.1016/j.gie.2009.10.047.
96. Kavitt RT, Ates F, Slaughter JC, et al. Randomized controlled trial comparing esophageal dilation to no dilation among adults with esophageal eosinophilia and dysphagia. Dis Esophagus. 2015;29:983–91. https://doi.org/10.1111/dote.12398.
97. Runge TM, Eluri S, Cotton CC, et al. Causes and outcomes of esophageal perforation in eosinophilic esophagitis. J Clin Gastroenterol. 2016;51:805–13. https://doi.org/10.1097/MCG.0000000000000718.
98. Cohen MS, Kaufman AB, Palazzo JP, Nevin D, Dimarino AJ Jr, Cohen S. An audit of endoscopic complications in adult eosinophilic esophagitis. Clin Gastroenterol Hepatol. 2007;5(10):1149–53. https://doi.org/10.1016/j.cgh.2007.05.017.
99. Schoepfer AM, Gonsalves N, Bussmann C, et al. Esophageal dilation in eosinophilic esophagitis: effectiveness, safety, and impact on the underlying inflammation. Am J Gastroenterol. 2010;105(5):1062–70. https://doi.org/10.1038/ajg.2009.657.
100. Jacobs JW Jr, Spechler SJ. A systematic review of the risk of perforation during esophageal dilation for patients with eosinophilic esophagitis. Dig Dis Sci. 2010;55(6):1512–5. https://doi.org/10.1007/s10620-010-1165-x.

MIX
Papier aus verantwortungsvollen Quellen
Paper from responsible sources
FSC® C105338

If you have any concerns about our products,
you can contact us on
ProductSafety@springernature.com

In case Publisher is established outside the EU,
the EU authorized representative is:
Springer Nature Customer Service Center GmbH
Europaplatz 3, 69115 Heidelberg, Germany

Printed by Libri Plureos GmbH
in Hamburg, Germany